VOLUME 582   JULY 2002

THE ANNALS

of The American Academy *of* Political
and Social Science

ROBERT PEARSON, *Executive Editor*
ALAN W. HESTON, *Editor*

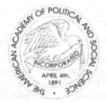

CROSS-NATIONAL
DRUG POLICY

Special Editors of this Volume

ROBERT MacCOUN
University of California, Berkeley
PETER REUTER
University of Maryland

SAGE Publications   *THOUSAND OAKS   LONDON   NEW DELHI*

The American Academy of Political and Social Science

c/o Fels Center of Government, University of Pennsylvania, 3814 Walnut Street, Philadelphia, PA 19104; (215) 746-6500; (215) 898-1202 (fax); www.1891.org

---

Origin and Purpose. The Academy was organized December 14, 1889, to promote the progress of political and social science, especially through publications and meetings. The Academy does not take sides in controverted questions, but seeks to gather and present reliable information to assist the public in forming an intelligent and accurate judgment.

Meetings. The Academy occasionally holds a meeting in the spring extending over two days.

Publications. THE ANNALS of the American Academy of Political and Social Science is the bimonthly publication of The Academy. Each issue contains articles on some prominent social or political problem, written at the invitation of the editors. Also, monographs are published from time to time, numbers of which are distributed to pertinent professional organizations. These volumes constitute important reference works on the topics with which they deal, and they are extensively cited by authorities throughout the United States and abroad. The papers presented at the meetings of The Academy are included in THE ANNALS.

Membership. Each member of The Academy receives THE ANNALS and may attend the meetings of The Academy. Membership is open only to individuals. Annual dues: $65.00 for the regular paperbound edition (clothbound, $100.00). For members outside the U.S.A., add $24.00 for shipping of your subscription. Members may also purchase single issues of THE ANNALS for $20.00 each (clothbound, $28.00).

Subscriptions. THE ANNALS of the American Academy of Political and Social Science (ISSN 0002-7162) is published six times annually—in January, March, May, July, September, and November—by Sage Publications, 2455 Teller Road, Thousand Oaks, CA 91320. Telephone: (800) 818-SAGE (7243) and (805) 499-9774; FAX/Order line: (805) 499-0871. Copyright © 2002 by the American Academy of Political and Social Science. Institutions may subscribe to THE ANNALS at the annual rate: $420.00 (clothbound, $475.00). Add $24.00 per year for subscriptions outside the U.S.A. Institutional rates for single issues: $81.00 each (clothbound, $91.00).

Periodicals postage paid at Thousand Oaks, California, and at additional mailing offices.

Single issues of THE ANNALS may be obtained by individuals who are not members of The Academy for $32.00 each (clothbound, $42.00). Single issues of THE ANNALS have proven to be excellent supplementary texts for classroom use. Direct inquiries regarding adoptions to THE ANNALS c/o Sage Publications (address below).

All correspondence concerning membership in The Academy, dues renewals, inquiries about membership status, and/or purchase of single issues of THE ANNALS should be sent to THE ANNALS c/o Sage Publications, 2455 Teller Road, Thousand Oaks, CA 91320. Telephone: (800) 818-SAGE (7243) and (805) 499-9774; FAX/Order line: (805) 499-0871. *Please note that orders under $30 must be prepaid.* Sage affiliates in London and India will assist institutional subscribers abroad with regard to orders, claims, and inquiries for both subscriptions and single issues.

THE ANNALS

© 2002 *by* The American Academy *of* Political *and* Social Science

Editorial Office: Fels Center of Government, University of Pennsylvania, 3814 Walnut Street, Philadelphia, PA 19104-6197.

For information about membership* (individuals only) and subscriptions (institutions), address:

SAGE PUBLICATIONS
2455 Teller Road
Thousand Oaks, CA 91320

Sage Production Staff: BARBARA CORRIGAN, SCOTT SPRINGER, and ROSE TYLAK

From India and South Asia, *write to:*		*From Europe, the Middle East,* *and Africa, write to:*
SAGE PUBLICATIONS INDIA Pvt. Ltd		SAGE PUBLICATIONS LTD
P.O. Box 4215		6 Bonhill Street
New Delhi 110 048		London EC2A 4PU
INDIA		UNITED KINGDOM

*Please note that members of The Academy receive THE ANNALS with their membership.
International Standard Serial Number ISSN 0002-7162
International Standard Book Number ISBN 0-7619-2744-1 (Vol. 582, 2002 paper)
International Standard Book Number ISBN 0-7619-2743-3 (Vol. 582, 2002 cloth)
First printing, July 2002.

The articles appearing in THE ANNALS are abstracted or indexed in *Academic Abstracts, Academic Search, America: History and Life, Asia Pacific Database, Book Review Index, CAB Abstracts Database, Central Asia: Abstracts & Index, Communication Abstracts, Corporate ResourceNET, Criminal Justice Abstracts, Current Citations Express, Current Contents: Social & Behavioral Sciences, e-JEL, EconLit, Expanded Academic Index, Guide to Social Science & Religion in Periodical Literature, Health Business FullTEXT, HealthSTAR FullTEXT, Historical Abstracts, International Bibliography of the Social Sciences, International Political Science Abstracts, ISI Basic Social Sciences Index, Journal of Economic Literature on CD, LEXIS-NEXIS, MasterFILE FullTEXT, Middle East: Abstracts & Index, North Africa: Abstracts & Index, PAIS International, Periodical Abstracts, Political Science Abstracts, Sage Public Administration Abstracts, Social Science Source, Social Sciences Citation Index, Social Sciences Index Full Text, Social Services Abstracts, Social Work Abstracts, Sociological Abstracts, Southeast Asia: Abstracts & Index, Standard Periodical Directory (SPD), TOPICsearch, Wilson OmniFile V,* and *Wilson Social Sciences Index/Abstracts,* and are available on microfilm from University Microfilms, Ann Arbor, Michigan.

Information about membership rates, institutional subscriptions, and back issue prices may be found on the facing page.

Advertising. Current rates and specifications may be obtained by writing to THE ANNALS Advertising and Promotion Manager at the Thousand Oaks office (address above).

Claims. Claims for undelivered copies must be made no later than six months following month of publication. The publisher will supply missing copies when losses have been sustained in transit and when the reserve stock will permit.

Change of Address. Six weeks' advance notice must be given when notifying of change of address to ensure proper identification. Please specify name of journal. **POSTMASTER:** Send address changes to: THE ANNALS of the American Academy of Political and Social Science, c/o Sage Publications, 2455 Teller Road, Thousand Oaks, CA 91320.

THE ANNALS

of The American Academy *of* Political
and Social Science

ROBERT PEARSON, *Executive Editor*
ALAN W. HESTON, *Editor*

--------------- FORTHCOMING ---------------

ALTERNATIVE MEDICINES
Special Editors: Helen Scheehan
and Barry Brenton

Volume 583   September 2002

HEALTH AND THE ENVIRONMENT
Special Editor: Phil Brown

Volume 584   November 2002

HIGHER EDUCATION IN THE
TWENTY-FIRST CENTURY
Special Editor: Paul Rich

Volume 585   January 2003

See page 2 for information on Academy membership and
purchase of single volumes of **The Annals.**

CONTENTS

The Varieties of Drug Control at the Dawn of the Twenty-First Century

The world now has a century of experience with refined cocaine and heroin and has observed their consequences. For most of that century, as many citizens in the industrialized nations experimented with those drugs, their governments experimented with various forms of legal prohibition. A few countries—most notably the Netherlands, Great Britain, and Switzerland—have been willing to test a wide range of control strategies. Most others—including the United States—have generally tinkered at the margins of a narrow criminal justice model, perhaps augmented with minimal provision of public drug treatment.

Some foreign experiences have long been a staple of the American drug debate—most notably the British experience with prescription heroin in the mid-twentieth century and Dutch de facto cannabis legalization since the late 1970s. In the absence of careful scholarly description, U.S. observers have been free to characterize such experiences in whichever way serves their rhetorical purposes. For example, a rapid increase in the minimal base rate of heroin use in Britain in the late 1960s became the basis for a charge that the British system of heroin prescription had failed; we discuss below a more reasonable interpretation of this experience.

Only recently have scholars, policy analysts, and policy makers from different nations begun to look outside their own boundaries to see what might be learned from experiences abroad (e.g., Estievenart 1995; MacCoun and Reuter 2001a, 2001b; Reuband 1995).

This special issue describes the experiences of eleven nations: Australia, Canada, Colombia, Denmark, France, Iran, Jamaica, Mexico, Portugal, Russia, and Sweden. Each of these countries is confronting the various public health and public safety problems caused both by domestic drug consumption and by the legal prohibition of these substances. Some countries confront a second drug problem as well, one that can dwarf the first: they are home to major drug trafficking organizations. And several of these countries must contend with the direct and indirect effects of an aggressive U.S. campaign to stem the flow of drugs.

THE PITFALLS OF CROSS-NATIONAL DRUG POLICY ANALYSIS

The obstacles to rigorous cross-national comparative work are daunting in any domain, but particularly so for psychoactive drug use because of its illicit and heavily stigmatized nature. Indeed, no other nation comes close to the

United States with respect to the breadth and depth of its measurement of drug use and drug-related problems, and yet a recent National Academy of Science panel found the state of U.S. drug policy assessment and analysis to be quite inadequate for making informed decisions (Manski, Pepper, and Petrie 2001). (Whether American politicians would actually avail themselves of better information is an open question; see Schecter 2002 [this issue]; MacCoun 2001.)

There are four basic analytical challenges for cross-national drug policy analysis:

Data scarcity. With respect to the prevalence and incidence of illicit drug use, few nations have anything comparable to the federally funded National Household Survey on Drug Abuse (posted annually at http://www.samhsa. gov/oas/nhsda.htm) and the University of Michigan's Monitoring the Future annual high school senior survey (posted annually at http:// monitoringthefuture.org/) in the United States. Until recently, only the Netherlands and a few isolated cities had anything more than occasional ad hoc prevalence surveys. As a result, until recently, there were few years in which any more than a handful of national estimates were available for comparison (see MacCoun and Reuter 2001a). Time series are almost nonexistent. The creation of the European Monitoring Center on Drugs and Drug Abuse has brought major improvements, but the series still cover only a few years.

Poor data quality and comparability. Existing drug data series are rarely created for research purposes but instead reflect the activities of various public and private agencies—police arrests, court sanctions, customs seizures, and emergency room overdoses (Manski, Pepper, and Petrie 2001). As such, they are neither pure measures of drug prevalence nor unambiguous indicators of policy preference. Making matters worse, similar bureaucracies in different nations rarely adopt the same definitions of such seemingly basic concepts as drug-related death, drug possession arrest, and so on. For example, French medical examiners are much more reluctant to classify a death as drug related than are German medical examiners. Whether through duplicity or incompetence, American commentators routinely compare data on, say, Dutch versus U.S. marijuana use without equating the years, age ranges, or question wording underlying the estimates. Indeed, our own efforts to produce defensibly comparable cross-national estimates of marijuana use have been controversial (see MacCoun 2001, MacCoun and Reuter 2001b, and the correspondence section of the *British Journal of Psychiatry* throughout 2001).

There are reasons to believe these data problems will become less severe in the coming years. Cross-national work in drug policy is being facilitated by increasingly sophisticated data collection and coordination efforts, including the World Health Organization's European survey of drug use among school children (Hibell et al. 1997), the Pompidou Group's multicity study (Hartnoll 1994), and especially the periodic monographs assembled by the European Monitoring Centre for Drugs and Drug Addiction (2000).

Weak causal inference. Finally, even where suitable data exist, correlational evidence provides only weak evidence on the consequences of drug policies (Manski, Pepper, and Petrie 2001; Shadish, Cook, and Campbell 2001). Making matters seemingly worse, the paucity of strong time-series data largely preclude rigorous econometric analyses. Yet we would argue that an acknowledgement of the necessity of weak causal inference hardly implies that nothing can be learned. Later in this article, we will attempt to explicate some of the alternative and reciprocal pathways linking cultures, drug policies, and drug-related outcomes.

Unknown generalizability. We stipulate that nations and cultures differ in myriad ways, making cross-national generalization hazardous. This problem differs from that confronting within-nation research (across jurisdictions, settings, investigators, and periods) in degree rather than kind—external validity is always uncertain in policy research (Shadish, Cook, and Campbell 2001). It is too easy to simply reject cross-national evidence out of hand when one dislikes the conclusions. The important analytic question is, When does a difference truly make a difference?

Arguably, generalizing from historical evidence on drug policy is more problematic than generalizing across modern cultures. Surely the sociological distance between the United States of 1910 and the United States of today is in many ways larger than the current cultural gap separating the Netherlands, Sweden, and the United States. Most industrialized nations experienced major drug epidemics in the 1970s or 1980s, triggered perhaps by Western counterculture but later fueled by the development of increasingly large-scale and sophisticated trafficking networks. The sheer scale of the modern problem weakens the relevance of preepidemic historical analogies. The British heroin prescription regime of the mid-twentieth century provides an illustration (MacCoun and Reuter 2001a, chap. 12). Many Americans have noted that the British made heroin legally available before 1967. In support of legalization, some then cite the rarity of heroin addiction during most of that period. Critics respond by citing the large percentage increase in the addict rate when a few doctors began reckless prescribing. But in fact there is much less here than meets the eye. The pre-1967 regime was not legalization, and not, in legal terms, very different from what replaced it. The growth that led to the 1967 change involved in absolute terms only a few hundred heroin users. Britain's major heroin epidemic occurred much later and—as noted above—was not unlike that experienced in other industrialized nations.

THE BENEFITS OF CROSS-NATIONAL DRUG POLICY ANALYSIS

Despite these obvious barriers to rigorous analysis, we see a great value in more cross-national work. There are vigorous debates about the future of drug policy in the United States, Canada, Latin America, Europe, and the Antipodes. The options under debate include the perennial budgetary battles between supply and demand reduction efforts but also more dramatic possibilities such as medical marijuana, decriminalization, commercial legalization, heroin maintenance, and a range of harm reduction interventions. Elsewhere, we review the available theory and evidence for these options in detail (MacCoun and Reuter 2001a).

Confident policy forecasting is precluded by the absence of a strong theoretical foundation. Though glib pronouncements are frequently made on the basis of simple back-of-the-envelope economic models, these analyses are almost certainly crude caricatures of the reality of drug markets. We know far too little about the structural relationships among relevant variables or the relevant parameters (see Caulkins and Reuter 1998; Manski, Pepper, and Petrie 2001). For example, until fairly recently, it was assumed without evidence that hard-drug addicts are quite insensitive to price—in economic jargon, it was thought that demand was relatively price inelastic. Recent estimates have seriously challenged this view, at least for cocaine (Caulkins and Reuter 1998).

And progress in such debates is hindered by what social scientists would call restricted range in the independent variable—few nations have experimented with enough policy variations to learn much from their own experiences. But cross-national comparisons reveal that radical new ideas in one country are sometimes old hat in another. Heroin prescription regimes are one example. The recent Swiss trials in heroin maintenance are more innovative in their scope and design, but there are several precedents: the British experience discussed above, a brief flirtation with heroin prescription in Sweden in the 1960s (Lenke and Olsson 2002 [this issue]), and even Iran's program of opium ration coupons in the early twentieth century (Raisdana 2002 [this issue]).

All the nations discussed in this issue have adopted some form of legal prohibition against drugs such as cannabis, cocaine, heroin, and the psychedelics. Indeed, each of the nations is a signatory to the major international treaties requiring them to prohibit recreational use of heroin, cocaine, and marijuana. The treaties are the 1961 Single Convention on Narcotic Substances, the 1971 Convention on Psychotropic Substances, and the 1988 Convention against Illicit Trafficking in Narcotic Drugs and Psychotropic Substances (see Estievenart 1995). These documents have probably played some role in constraining national legal experimentation.

The Dutch cannabis regime is the only contemporary model that approximates legalization of a major recreational drug currently banned in the United States. Despite its de jure cannabis prohibition, the Netherlands has adopted a formal nonprosecution policy for possession and sale of less than five grams of cannabis, and cannabis is widely available for retail sale in Dutch coffee shops and in some nightclubs (MacCoun and Reuter 2001b). Nonetheless, cannabis is formally illicit, and the production and wholesale distribution of cannabis are subject to significant enforcement activities.

Despite the universality of drug prohibition, there are important variations in the aggressiveness of legal sanctioning against drug possession and drug use. Spain and Italy have "depenalized"—a term we prefer to the more ambiguous "decriminalized"—possession of all street drugs. In various degrees, the Netherlands, parts of Australia, the United States, and Germany have depenalized marijuana possession. Portugal (van het Loo, van Beusekom, and Kahan 2002 [this issue]), Switzerland, and most recently, England are in the process of doing the same. Nations also differ in their formal treatment policies, including the availability and accessibility of public treatment and of methadone maintenance. Drug treatment can seem like a more tolerant alternative to criminal justice sanctioning, but there is a concern with net widening both here and abroad (see Covington 2001). Court-mandated treatment is an increasingly common alternative to traditional drug sentencing in the United States (and is being extended in California to be the only possible sentence for some categories of offenders), but Sweden is distinctive in its use of mandatory treatment even for those not formally prosecuted for a drug offense.

A dozen U.S. states have decriminalized marijuana possession to some extent, and simple cross-sectional and longitudinal analyses in the United States and Australia suggest no impact on marijuana prevalence. Needle exchanges have been evaluated fairly rigorously in the United States and several other countries, with favorable results. Italy offers an intriguing natural experiment in hard-drug decriminalization, having decriminalized possession in the mid-1970s, recriminalized possession in 1990, and redecriminalized possession in 1993. Alas, the paucity of prevalence data renders the resulting experiences highly ambiguous. (See MacCoun and Reuter 2001a.)

ANALYTIC FRAMEWORK

As an overview to the articles of this special issue, we offer in Figure 1 a general analytical framework for thinking through the complex set of causal relationships among cultures, governments, drug policies, drug use, and drug outcomes (see MacCoun and Reuter 2001a, chap. 10). Our hope is that the framework, once articulated, will seem obvious, though the principles we articulate here are routinely overlooked or ignored in drug policy debates on both sides of the Atlantic. It is tempting to think in terms of a simple causal chain: goals → policies → implementation → prevalence of drug use → prevalence of drug harms. Figure 1 suggests that the situation is almost certainly more complex.

FIGURE 1
ANALYTIC FRAMEWORK LINKING DRUG POLICIES AND OUTCOMES

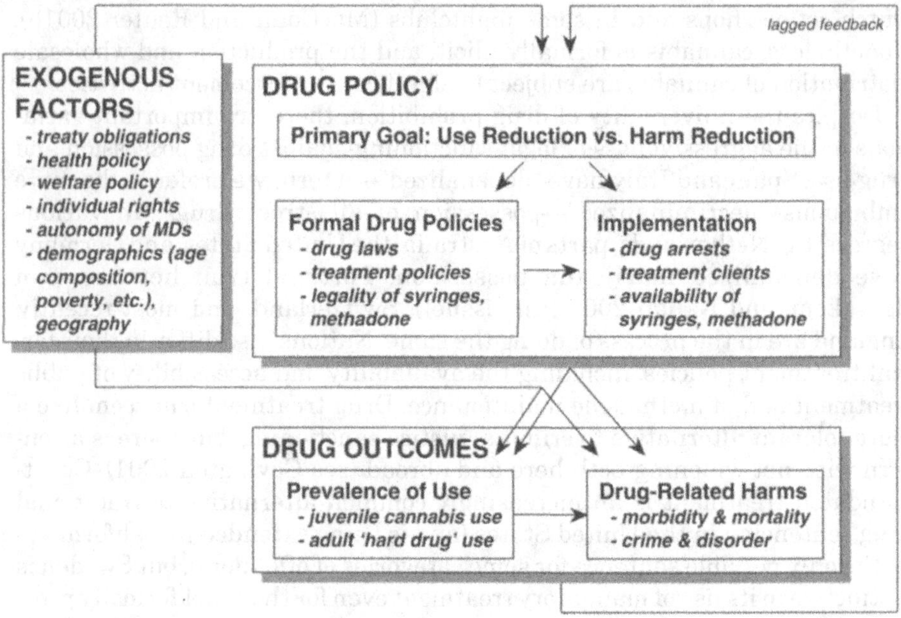

Four points stand out. First, many exogenous factors influence both drug policy and drug outcomes: international treaties, health and welfare policies, individual rights, the authority and autonomy of physicians, and sociodemographics. Second, goals directly influence not only formal policies but also their implementation. Indeed, in some nations (most notably the Netherlands), implementation more closely reflects national goals than do formal drug laws. Third, formal policies have symbolic influences that transcend the intensity of their implementation; they make moral statements and thus influence the perceived fairness and legitimacy of authorities, which in turn influences compliance. Fourth, formal policies and their implementation each have a direct influence on drug-related harms that may be largely independent of their effects on levels of drug use. This is the central insight of the European harm reduction movement. And finally, prevalence and harms have a lagged feedback effect on drug policy; for example, European drug policies have evolved considerably during the past two decades in response to a heroin epidemic (beginning in the 1970s) and an AIDS epidemic (surfacing in the 1980s). A liberal policy in a nation with a severe drug problem may be a response to perceived failure of an earlier, more repressive, policy. That the problem remains severe is not necessarily a failure of that new policy but perhaps a reflection of the intractability of severe drug addiction in a cohort of longtime users. Preventing a worsening of that problem may itself be a significant accomplishment.

Measuring the extent of a nation's drug problem requires more than estimating the number of persons using illicit drugs. Drugs differ in the damage that they cause users (e.g., cocaine's acute and chronic harms are greater than those of cannabis) and in the damage that their users cause to the rest of society. There may also be differences in the ways in which the drugs are used, which would have important consequences for the extent of harms suffered by users. For example, many Dutch addicts have long preferred smoking heroin to injecting it, a cultural norm that surely helped reduce HIV transmission in the 1990s.

We give particular emphasis to the many exogenous factors that influence both drug policy and drug outcomes: international treaties, health and welfare policies, individual rights, the authority and autonomy of physicians, and sociodemographics. The articles in this issue provide many examples.

The word "culture" can too easily become a fig leaf hiding our naked ignorance of the epidemiology of recreational drugs, but there is little doubt that broader social trends shape both drug use and drug policies. The countercultural movements of the 1960s and the 1970s (the hippies, the yippies, the Provos, and so on) have been noted already. Other examples include the Swedish alcohol temperance movement (Lenke and Olsson 2002), the breakdown of the Soviet Union (Paoli 2002 [this issue]), and the Islamic revolution in Iran (Raisdana 2002).

Choices are also clearly influenced by political values and definitions of what constitutes the drug problem. American commentators have long parsed the topic of drug policy into two competing visions: public health versus criminal justice, with the former approvingly cited as a more tolerant alternative to the American predeliction for the latter. There is clearly a large grain of truth to this scheme. No country in Europe experiences anything remotely approaching the criminal violence associated with the drug trade in the United States. So it is perhaps understandable that Americans, uniquely among citizens of rich nations, have largely construed the problem as one of crime control. Mexico (Chabat 2002 [this issue]), Colombia (Thoumi 2002 [this issue]), and Jamaica (Jones 2002 [this issue]) do have very high levels of drug-related violence, and violence does indeed figure prominently in the debates about drugs in those nations.

Yet European experiences suggest that the opposite pole—the public health perspective—is far from being a homogeneous category and indeed is hardly incompatible with cultural intolerance. The Swiss have been more willing than almost anyone to experiment with medical alternatives to prison for opiate addicts, yet they also have the highest drug arrest rates in Western Europe (MacCoun and Reuter 2001a, chap. 10). Sweden is, by European standards, remarkably intolerant in its antidrug rhetoric and its drug laws, yet it is more generous than the tolerant Dutch in its investment in services for drug addicts. According to Gould (1988),

from an Anglo-Saxon point of view, we may shrink from the coercive measures and il-
liberal controls the Swedes are prepared to adopt, but on the positive side it can be said
that they show more concern than we do over the damage people do to themselves
through the consumption of alcohol and the taking of drugs. (P. 127)

Nations also differ in their traditions of physician autonomy and authority.
In Britain, the relative power of the medical profession and its determination
to allow physicians full autonomy has probably been the principal explanation for the continuation of the right to prescribe heroin to addicted patients.
Lenke and Olsson (2002) and Bergeron and Kopp (2002 [this issue]) discuss
changes in the attitudes of Swedish and French physicians, respectively, toward their proper role in illicit drug problems.

The vagaries of geography are another example of important exogenous
factors. In his masterful book *Guns, Germs, and Steel*, Jared Diamond (1997)
argued persuasively for the dramatic and largely underestimated role that
purely geographic factors—ease of transit, climate, flora, and fauna—have
played in the shaping of world history. The history of drug consumption and
production provides ample illustrations. In this special issue, Chabat,
Thoumi, and Jones each discuss the role of local climate on drug cultivation in
Mexico, Colombia, and Jamaica, respectively.

Location relative to major markets also influences problems and policies.
Mexico has been called a "natural smuggling platform" for the United States,
while Colombia's role as principal heroin producer to the U.S. market is also a
consequence of the ease of shipment compared to cheaper producers such as
Afghanistan and Myanmar. Jamaica is an attractive supplement to Mexico
for transshipment purposes. Iran is yet another nation cursed by location.
Though not close to large and rich consumer markets, it has been for the past
decade the most convenient route for the export of Afghan heroin to Western
Europe. Elsewhere, we discuss other examples, including the distinctive
spread of HIV among injection drug users across Southern Europe or the
influence of Rotterdam's international port in shaping the Netherlands' dominant role in European drug interdiction statistics (MacCoun and Reuter
2001a).

Most notably, several authors identify the United States, especially U.S.
drug control officials, as a major exogenous force shaping their own nations'
drug policies (e.g., Chabat 2002 on Mexico; Thoumi 2002 on Colombia;
Laursen and Jepsen 2002 on Denmark; Bammer and colleagues 2002 [this
issue] on Australia). Indeed, this is the central theme of the articles by Jones
(2002) on Jamaica and by Schecter (2002) on U.S. misrepresentation of Canadian needle-exchange research findings. But the United States is not unique
in its international lobbying role. For example, Laursen and Jepsen (2002
[this issue]) cite Swedish efforts to influence Danish drug policy. And the
Netherlands has been under enormous pressure to "harmonize" its drug policies with those of other European Union states (MacCoun and Reuter 2001a,
chap. 11).

OVERVIEW OF THE ARTICLES

We have organized the articles into three sections, by geography and wealth.

The wealthy West

The first section describes the problems and responses of wealthy Western nations with respect to a variety of drug problems that have generally worsened since the 1960s. Lau Laursen and Jorgen Jepsen (2002) chronicle the evolution of Denmark's drug policy during a thirty-year period, characterizing it as highly ambivalent, a mix of soft rhetoric at the political level and conservative policies in practice. Though there are some pragmatic innovations that could be characterized as harm reduction, such as the creation of a free marijuana sales zone in the Christiana neighborhood of Copenhagen and the liberal dispensation of methadone, these do not come from any clearly articulated vision of drug policy.

This contrasts sharply with the experience of Sweden, as summarized by Leif Lenke and Boerje Olsson (2002). Though there have been brief periods of experimentation, most notably with maintenance programs for methamphetamine users and heroin users in the 1960s, Sweden's policy has had a consistently repressive character, supported by powerful nongovernmental organizations and professional groups. Rates of drug use and drug-related problems have been notably low relative to other European nations during a long period; there is vigorous debate about how much this reflects the tough policy.

France and Portugal are of particular interest because each has recently seen sharp changes in drug policy in recent years, each with its own dynamic. Henri Bergeron and Pierre Kopp (2002) describe the role of French health professionals in overcoming long ideological resistance to any but an abstinence philosophy. In a very short period in the mid-1990s, they promoted and developed a system of treatment based on maintenance of heroin addicts on methadone and a relatively new drug, buprenorphine. Although it is too early to judge its success, this new policy has produced huge increases in the number of users in treatment. In Portugal, as chronicled by Mirjam van het Loo and colleagues (2002), professional opinion also played a decisive role. In this case, a commission of experts from a variety of backgrounds were asked to provide recommendations to deal with the rising use of drugs, particularly heroin. The commission developed an explicit harm reduction approach, which was then the basis for a sweeping legislation that went into effect in 2001; no outcome results are available.

Australia is the most explicitly harm reductionist nation among those discussed in this issue. Gabriele Bammer and colleagues (2002) describe a policy that has, even in the face of rapidly increasing heroin deaths and other drug-related problems, maintained programs aimed at helping users cope with their problems. Yet enforcement has been aggressive, and there has been resistance to a number of harm reduction interventions (safe injecting rooms, trials of heroin maintenance).

The western hemisphere

For three of the nations discussed in this issue (Colombia, Jamaica, and Mexico), U.S. consumption and U.S. international policies are the dominant realities both for policy making and in the generation of problems. Mexico has served as a principal foreign source of the major U.S. drugs for decades. Not only does it produce much of the heroin, methamphetamine, and marijuana consumed in the United States but it has for at least a decade served as the primary transshipment route for cocaine from the Andes. Jorge Chabat (2002) describes how this has created newly violent and powerful criminal groups, even though Mexican drug use remains at modest levels. Mexican policy makers, facing the wrath of a dominant neighbor, have had little room for flexibility in policy making.

What U.S.-destined cocaine is not shipped through Mexico comes through the Caribbean, and Jamaica plays a particularly prominent role. Marlyn Jones (2002) describes how drug trafficking has exacerbated the long-standing problem of politically related gang violence by increasing both the moneys and the weapons involved. Again, the United States looms as the dominant external political force pushing for aggressive enforcement, with decertification and both financial and immigration sanctions as powerful weapons.

Colombia is the principal production source of cocaine and (more recently) heroin for the United States. Francisco Thoumi (2002) relates this role to the chronic instability of Colombia, a long tradition of international smuggling, and a lack of civil society. The large earnings from the cocaine trade have again exacerbated the political violence by increasing the financial stakes. U.S. pressure for extradition of major traffickers has forced the Colombian government to enact legislation that in the late 1980s led to the most serious attack by criminal groups on central government. Drug use is a relatively minor concern of Colombian drug policy; instead, policy has been focused on trafficking and related corruption and violence.

The transition countries

Iran and Russia present the case of nations in transition in many senses. Letizia Paoli (2002) chronicles the development of a new drug problem in Russia, following the collapse of the Soviet Union. In 1990, Russia had a very modest level of drug use, primarily supplied domestically. By the end of the decade, it had been fully integrated into the international drug market, particularly for heroin, and indicators of drug use and problems had soared. The policy response has been highly intolerant. Even legislation aimed at emphasizing treatment for drug possession offenses has largely been subverted to allow the police maximum power over arrested drug users. There is little political debate around the issue in the midst of a period of fundamental economic and social change.

Iran has a much longer history of dealing with opiate abuse. Fariborz Raisdana, in collaboration with Ahmad Gharavi Nakhjavani (2002), shows how Iran has struggled throughout the twentieth century to deal with a very salient problem of opiate addiction and trafficking. Policies have shifted frequently between harsh punishment and efforts to regulate use of heroin and opium. The Islamic revolution of 1978 brought to power a government employing draconian punishments of both users and sellers. Faced with a continued high rate of addiction, the past decade has seen experimentation with much more therapeutically oriented approaches. At the same time, notwithstanding aggressive border enforcement, Iran has suffered from its role as the main transit country for heroin exiting from Afghanistan on the way to Europe.

Two articles are not country specific. Martin Schechter (2002) describes how politicians in the United States knowingly and extensively distorted the results of a major study of needle exchange in Vancouver. His article illustrates graphically how much the United States stands out from other nations in the aggressiveness and politicization of drug policies.

Finally, money laundering controls, the subject of Michael Levi's (2002 [this issue]) article, represent the ultimate instance of international interdependence centered on drug policy. A new regulatory regime has been created that governs the banking systems of almost all developed nations, justified by the belief that illegal drugs account for a substantial fraction of suspicious financial transactions, particularly across national borders. Total money seizures from this system, though large in absolute terms, are minimal when compared to the (probably inflated) estimates of world drug expenditures. Money laundering controls may serve other purposes well, particularly in the new fight against international terrorism, but are unlikely to do much to reduce drug problems.

CONCLUSIONS

As so often is the case with cross-national comparisons, one learns first what is feasible. The Dutch have shown that harm reduction can be used as a principle to consistently guide decisions, and have some successes to show and no disasters to hide. Portugal's sudden shift to harm reduction (van het Loo, van Beusekom, and Kahan 2002) will allow testing of whether the Dutch experience represents something idiosyncratic about the Netherlands. Denmark has experience with liberal prescription of methadone (Laursen and Jepsen 2002), which may be highly relevant as the United States considers relaxation of its current tough regulation of opiate maintenance. The Swiss trials show that heroin maintenance programs can operate in an orderly and systematic fashion for the benefit of a substantial fraction of the clients.

These ought to be important facts for drug policy debates in the United States.

But even societies less similar to the United States than those of Western Europe can provide useful insights. U.S. policies toward Jamaica and Mexico impose a high cost; wrapped in moralistic rhetoric, they force on these nations the burden of dealing with American problems. Understanding what these nations might do if they were given their own options and could focus on the welfare of their own citizens would help the United States to act as a better citizen in the world. Iran's experiences with different regulatory regimes aimed at allowing use for those already addicted while suppressing the black market could, with more data, contribute to discussion of different options within a general prohibition framework.

Drug policy, as we have suggested throughout this article, is the result of many forces. A better understanding of what has been tried elsewhere and what has come of it should be one influence.

ROBERT MacCOUN

PETER REUTER

References

Bammer, G., W. Hall, M. Hamilton, and R. Ali. 2002. Harm minimization in a prohibition context—Australia. *Annals of the American Academy of Political and Social Science* 582:80-93.

Bergeron, H., and P. Kopp. 2002. Policy paradigms, ideas, and interests: The case of the French public health policy toward drug abuse. *Annals of the American Academy of Political and Social Science* 582:37-49.

Caulkins, J., and P. Reuter. 1998. What can we learn from drug prices? *Journal of Drug Issues* 28 (3): 593-612.

Chabat, J. 2002. Mexico's war on drugs: No margin for maneuver. *Annals of the American Academy of Political and Social Science* 582:134-48.

Covington, J. 2001. Linking treatment to punishment: An evaluation of drug treatment in the criminal justice system. In *Informing America's policy on illegal drugs: What we don't know keeps hurting us*, edited by C. Manski, J. Pepper, and C. Petrie, 349-81. Washington, DC: National Academy of Sciences.

Diamond, J. 1997. *Guns, germs, and steel: The fates of human societies.* New York: Norton.

Estievenart, G., ed. 1995. *Policies and strategies to combat drugs in Europe.* Dordrecht, the Netherlands: Martinus Nijhoff.

European Monitoring Centre for Drugs and Drug Addiction. 2000. *Annual report on the state of the drugs problem in the European Union, 1999.* Lisbon, Portugal: European Monitoring Centre for Drugs and Drug Addiction.

Gould, A. 1988. *Conflict and control in welfare policy: The Swedish experience.* London: Longman.

Hartnoll, R. 1994. *Multi-city study: Drug misuse trends in thirteen European cities.* Cooperation Group to Combat Drug Abuse and Illicit Trafficking in Drugs (Pompidou Group). Strasbourg, France: Council of Europe Press.

Hibell, B., B. Andersson, T. Bjarnason, A. Kokkevi, M. Morgan, and A. Narusk. 1997. *The 1995 ESPAD report: Alcohol and other drug use among students in 26 European countries.* Stockholm: Swedish Council for Information on Alcohol and Other Drugs, Council of Europe Pompidou Group.

Jones, M. J. 2002. Policy paradox: Implications of U.S. drug control policy for Jamaica. *Annals of the American Academy of Political and Social Science* 582:117-33.

Laursen, L., and J. Jepsen. 2002. Danish drug policy—An ambivalent balance between repression and welfare. *Annals of the American Academy of Political and Social Science* 582:20-36.

Lenke, L., and B. Olsson. 2002. Swedish drug policy in the twenty-first century: A policy model going astray. *Annals of the American Academy of Political and Social Science* 582:65-79.

Levi, M. 2002. Money laundering and its regulation. *Annals of the American Academy of Political and Social Science* 582:181-94.

MacCoun, R. J. 2001. American distortion of Dutch drug statistics. *Society* 38:23-26.

MacCoun, R., and P. Reuter. 2001a. *Drug war heresies: Learning from other vices, times and places.* New York: Cambridge University Press.

———. 2001b. Evaluating alternative cannabis regimes. *British Journal of Psychiatry* 178:123-28.

Manski, C., J. Pepper, and C. Petrie. 2001. *Informing America's policy on illegal drugs: What we don't know keeps hurting us.* Washington, DC: National Academy of Sciences.

Paoli, L. 2002. The price of freedom: Illegal drug markets and policies in post-Soviet Russia. *Annals of the American Academy of Political and Social Science* 582:167-80.

Raisdana, F., with A. G. Nakhjavani. 2002. The drug market in Iran. *Annals of the American Academy of Political and Social Science* 582:149-166.

Reuband, K. H. 1995. Drug use and drug policy in Western Europe: Epidemiological findings in a comparative perspective. *European Addiction Research* 1:32-41.

Schechter, M. T. 2002. Science, ideology, and needle exchange programs. *Annals of the American Academy of Political and Social Science* 582:94-101.

Shadish, W. R., T. D. Cook, and D. T. Campbell. 2001. *Experimental and quasi-experimental designs for generalized causal inference.* Boston: Houghton Mifflin.

Thoumi, F. E. 2002. Illegal drugs in Colombia: From illegal economic boom to social crisis. *Annals of the American Academy of Political and Social Science* 582:102-16.

van het Loo, M., I. van Beusekom, and J. P. Kahan. 2002. Decriminalization of drug use in Portugal: The development of a policy. *Annals of the American Academy of Political and Social Science* 582:50-64.

Danish Drug Policy—
An Ambivalent Balance
between Repression and Welfare

By LAU LAURSEN and JORGEN JEPSEN

ABSTRACT: This article maps recent developments in drug policy in Denmark: control, treatment, prevention, and harm reduction. Prevailing issues have been the introduction of a Danish heroin experiment, injection rooms and other harm reduction measures, moral panics around street level phenomena, and a renewed discussion of the relative roles of law enforcement and treatment/harm reduction. The power positions of the actors—police, politicians, administrators, and users' representatives—have shifted over time. A covert conflict between the Ministry of Social Affairs and the Ministry of Health has resulted in an uneasy balance on the political and policy level and confusion about guidelines and practices. There have been oscillations between optimism and pessimism in the law enforcement and treatment sectors. Ritualistic invocations of prohibition, prevention, and treatment coupled with ideological opposition have not been able to stem increasing acceptance of harm reduction—a modified version of the Scandinavian welfare approach.

Lau Laursen, Ph.D., was formerly employed at the Centre for Alcohol and Drug Research, University of Aarhus, and is now working as a private drug research consultant. He focused his Ph.D. on the construction of Danish drug control policy since 1965 and has published articles on Danish and Nordic alcohol and drug policy.

Jorgen Jepsen is an associate professor of criminology (emeritus) at the University of Aarhus. He was the chairman of the Danish Centre for Alcohol and Drug Research from 1992 to 2000. He is a former member of the Danish Narcotics Council and the author of several articles on drug control policy in Scandinavian and international contexts.

DENMARK has traditionally been seen as a primary example of the Nordic welfare states. Also in relation to the way the country handles drug problems, there have been grounds for expecting that welfare thinking would influence the drug policies of the country. From an American vantage point, Denmark has been seen as one of the more liberal countries in Western Europe, its policies more or less in line with the tolerant drug policies of Holland and Switzerland. This view, however, is only to a limited extent still true, as Denmark has in recent years approached the restrictiveness of hardliners of Sweden and the United States and has been increasingly influenced by the United Nations organs: the International Narcotics Control Board; the United Nations Commission on Narcotic Drugs; and its executive branch, the United Nations Office for Drug Control and Crime Prevention.

But the policies and the discourses around them have been multifaceted and not characterized by clarity of principles or strategies. Repeated public statements have indicated that Danish drug policy is a little of everything: police repression of the drug traffickers and the men behind them; prevention in the form of information and local intervention in problematic conditions; and treatment in the form of a mixture of public and private, of inpatient and outpatient services. Treatment strategies apply a number of different models—some involving drug-free treatment, others involving substitution therapies. Finally, some harm reduction measures come in the form of low-threshold services, mostly on a charitable basis.

There have been several attempts to get support for more radically liberal measures: proposals for heroin experiments on lines similar to the Swiss model, the installation of health rooms allowing addicts to inject under hygienic and less stressful conditions than in the streets, possible liberalization of cannabis regulation (Parliamentary Committees on Health and on Social Affairs 1998), and decriminalization of the possession of drugs for one's own consumption.

It is interesting that most of such proposals have rarely come to an outright decision based on principles. Several proposals for heroin experiments presented by a party to the Left have been dragged out by the government but ultimately defeated in parliament—to be reiterated later. Safe injection rooms have—on recommendation by the International Narcotics Control Board—been turned down by the Ministry of Health in a secret process of negotiation with Nordic colleagues but without an open debate in parliament (Jepsen 2001). Use per se has never been criminalized, but possession has been met with sanctions varying from warning and fine to imprisonment (depending on whether the drugs were assumed to be for the person's own use or for sale). Relative police passivity in recent years in relation to the open cannabis market in the free city of Christiania has meant that the market has been able to survive as the possibly largest open drug-dealing scene anywhere in the Western world (Jepsen 1996a).

These developments are results of the uneasy balance between repressive drug policies and policies based more on a welfare philosophy. The result is that no clear policy exists, different verbalizations of the goals of policy exist side by side, and proposals are advanced and shot down for fairly unclear reasons.

The newest governmental white paper on drug policy from 1994 (Justitsministeriet, Socialministeriet og Sundhedsministeriet 1994) clearly shows this ambivalent "wobble-course" when it comes to the definition of Danish drug strategy. In the white paper, it is said that

in to-day's Danish society we have legal intoxicants in sufficient amounts and variations the harmful effects of which we already fight hard to minimize. Society does not need any more legal intoxicants. Consequently there is no doubt that the goal of Danish drug policy must be maintained: Even though it must probably be viewed as unrealistic to create a society totally free of drug abuse, society must refuse legalization and continue its fight against abuse and dependence and for a minimization of the harms which drug abuse causes to the individual drug abuser and to society. (P. 24)

There are, in other words, limits to repression and limits to liberalization, but these limits are unclear and subject to constant oscillations. From a liberal viewpoint, one may be satisfied that Danish drug policy is not as harsh as its Swedish counterpart. And from a control-oriented view, one may be satisfied that liberalization

has not gone very far: penalties are fairly high, even though they are lower than those of the other Nordic countries (Laursen 1996). Police are active internationally as well as in the streets, and treatment innovations are kept within rather traditional bounds.

Looking at more recent developments in Nordic drug control policy, there are indications that the policies of the various Nordic countries are becoming increasingly repressive and that Denmark is now approaching the styles of Norway and Sweden while Finland is following up from a slow beginning (Kouvonen, Rosenqvist, and Skretting 2001), without this being the result of a fully debated political choice. Rather, it has been carried through behind the scenes as Denmark and its sister countries have gradually lessened their traditional welfare stance in favor of a war-on-drugs-like approach, American style (Jepsen 2001).

The following sections will look more closely at how this has come about. Given the tendencies of some countries in Central Europe to work in the direction of less repressive and more experimental drug policies, what is the probable balance between treatment, control, and harm reduction in future Danish drug policy?

As long as there is no support for an outright and well-formulated liberal policy along the lines of the Swiss and Dutch policies, the battle between repression and welfare seems likely to give priority to repression in actual practice, inasmuch as a liberal policy requires consistent political support whereas

repression seems to be able to survive no matter how inefficient and
harm producing it may be.

RECENT DEVELOPMENTS IN
DANISH DRUG CONSUMPTION
PATTERNS AND DRUG PROBLEMS

After several years in the sixties
and seventies when cannabis dominated the markets and the discourse
on drugs, it gradually subsided and
for many years was a drug mainly
cherished by the remains of the hippie cultures hibernating in Christiania and in small collectives around
the country. But since the mid-1990s,
it has reemerged as the most frequently used drug and has been getting increasing attention. The open
market in Christiania has formed a
steady source of supply in spite of
repeated—but mostly halfhearted—
attempts at uprooting it (Jepsen
1996a). Cannabis also has spread
around the country, and occasional
seizures of large shipments from
Morocco and elsewhere have indicated that a thriving traffic has been
going on underground. No police
effort has been able to stop this
influx.

Cannabis is without doubt the
most used illegal drug. Surveys on
drug prevalence have been conducted in a very scattered and unsys-
tematic way in Denmark, but some
trends can be located concerning the
development in cannabis use.

During the 1990s, one-third of the
adult population reported that they
had ever tried cannabis, and past
year prevalence was situated
between 5 and 7 percent. From different national and local surveys, it

TABLE 1

**USE OF CANNABIS AMONG YOUTH,
VARIOUS SURVEYS FROM 1983 TO 1999,
LIFETIME PREVALENCE
(IN PERCENTAGES)**

National/Local, Year	N	Girls	Boys	M
Local, 1983	—	—	—	8
Local, 1987	—	—	—	11
Local, 1989	—	—	—	13
National, 1990	—	—	—	17
Local, 1991	—	19	25	22
Local, 1993	1,395	15	16	15
National, 1995	2,545	16	21	18
Local, 1997	846	19	28	23
National, 1999	1,787	21	30	25

SOURCE: Sundhedsstyrelsen (2001d, 3).
NOTE: Dashes indicate that there is no specified information.

becomes clear that the use of cannabis has grown steadily since the
beginning of the 1980s (see Table 1).

The latest Danish results from the
1999 European School Survey indicate that 25 percent of pupils in the
ninth grade have ever tried cannabis.
This is an increase of 7 percent since
the former school survey in 1995.
Fourteen percent of the pupils report
use in the past year, and 5 percent in
the last month (Sundhedsstyrelsen
2001b, 16).

In the spring of 2001, media attention was given to a number of hash
clubs turning up in central locations
in the larger Danish cities, disguised
as activity centers or clubs with various pretences. They worried their
neighbors due to the clientele, part of
whom apparently have been motor-
cycle club members with ostenta-
tious vest colors; and they worried
traditional youth club leaders, as
many juveniles seem to prefer the

hash clubs to the traditional youth clubs. Repeated attempts to legalize or decriminalize cannabis officially or to turn the hash clubs into regulated coffee shops Amsterdam style have been turned down, to some extent with reference to reports of an increasing number of juveniles seeking treatment for cannabis-related problems. On the contrary, a law was passed in June 2001 that in effect outlawed the hash clubs on a model seemingly directed at inappropriate usage of rented space in general.

At the other end of the scale is a fairly stable but aging group of users of heroin, mostly in the form of heroin chloride used for injection. According to the latest attempt at estimating the size of the group of heavy drug users in need of social assistance, the group numbers around 14,000 on a national scale (Socialministeriet 1998; Sundhedsstyrelsen 2000), around one-half of them staying or living in Copenhagen. According to the European Monitoring Centre on Drugs and Drug Addiction (EMCDDA) (1999), the national prevalence estimate of problematic drug users in Denmark is set at 3.4 to 4.1 problematic drug users per 1,000 fifteen- to fifty-four-year-old inhabitants out of a total population of well above 5 million. These compare to, for example, 2.8 to 4.2 in Norway, 2.8 to 3.2 in Holland, 2.7 to 10.5 in the United Kingdom, and 1.7 to 3.7 in Germany. Such estimates must be taken with considerable reservation; however, these data from the EMCDDA study were based on common definitions, in contrast to earlier similar surveys.

The down-and-out junkies visible in the central parts of Copenhagen are injecting heroin in the open and seem unresponsive to any attempts at rehabilitation. Part of this group, up to one-third, may be enrolled in treatment in the Copenhagen municipal treatment system, where they get methadone maintenance treatment. Two-thirds of them are not currently in such contact. Some members of these subcultures apparently occasionally supplement or substitute their intravenous heroin use with cocaine, and some may be considered rather indiscriminate polydrug users, but most in this group clearly prefer heroin injection.

A general pattern of experimentation among young people has been observed as an increasingly dominant phenomenon connected to an increasingly liberal attitude toward drugs and experimentation (Sundhedsstyrelsen 2000). Imitation of the jet set—but with somewhat less cocaine, due to its higher price—involves the use of amphetamine, ecstasy, and other party drugs. In 1999, 0.5 percent of medium-aged youth (seventeen to nineteen years old) indicated a regular use of cocaine. More than 3 percent of youth ages sixteen to twenty-four have ever tried cocaine, which is the third most used drug in this age group. Next to hashish, amphetamine is the drug most often reported among Danish users. The proportion of fifteen- to sixteen-year-olds having ever tried amphetamine rose from 1 percent in 1991 to 4 percent in 1999. Persons appearing for treatment for the first time in 1999 evidence the highest proportion reporting amphetamine as their main drug (Sundhedssty-relsen 2001b, 43).

Most attention, however, has recently been given to the spread of the use of ecstasy. Ecstasy appears to have spread rapidly among very youthful dance partygoers. Three youthful users are reported to have died as a result of impurities of ecstasy pills or the consumption of extreme numbers of pills to experience powerful effects (Sundheds-styrelsen 2001c).

Repeated allegations in the media that ecstasy use—and concomitant death risk—was spreading rapidly among youthful partygoers led to official action in the form of designation of two counties as "model counties" to experiment with intervention against ecstasy among youth (Sundhedsministeriet 2000). A number of activities were introduced, but surveys from these and other counties revealed that only a limited proportion of youth in the counties had actual experience with ecstasy. Gradually, the scare—which might be termed a moral panic—subsided, and today only the more long-sighted work in the counties persists. The ecstasy scare is a good illustration of the propensity of a few powerful tabloid newspapers to blow up stories from the drug field and turn them into "scandals" that then immediately are presented to politicians, who in most cases feel forced to institute swift action—with little knowledge about the factual situation or the way the scare as such may influence the youth in question. For some Danish youth, the ecstasy scare may have had effects as marginalizing as

did the cannabis scare in the 1960s (Laursen Storgaard 2000).

Drug-related problems are considered some of the most severe social problems in the eyes of public opinion in Denmark. Drug-related deaths are an indicator of the drug problem, which is discussed intensively by authorities, politicians, and the media. In the beginning of the 1990s, the number of deaths caused by drug use rose dramatically from around 125 in the last years of the 1980s to around 275 in 1997. Thereafter, one could register stagnation and light decline to a relatively high level of 242 deaths in 1999.

The HIV/AIDS situation in the drug addict population has been under control for several years. The health authorities estimate that only 4 percent of this population is infected with HIV. In 1998, 211 new HIV cases were reported, of which only 6 percent were connected with intravenous drug use. In 1999, the numbers were 9 percent of 282 new cases (Sundhedsstyrelsen 2001a, 27). In comparison to this, various forms of hepatitis are a much larger problem; it is spreading epidemically and is a major threat to addicts' health. In past years, 90 percent of new cases of hepatitis C have been related to intravenous drug use (Sundheds-styrelsen 2001b, 37), and 80 percent of injecting drug users are estimated to be infected with hepatitis C.

THE DEVELOPMENT OF DANISH DRUG CONTROL POLICY

Use of illegal drugs as a social phenomenon in modern Danish industrialized welfare society developed during the 1960s. It first became visible as a cannabis culture, which was connected with the youth rebellion elements of protest against bourgeois lifestyle, but soon the cannabis problem was institutionalized as a social problem in Danish society.

In the beginning, authorities and the public looked at the cannabis problem as a question of social control, and development of drug control and police action were the measures society chose to use. In 1969, the maximum penalty for illegal handling of drugs was raised from imprisonment for two years to imprisonment for six years, while at the same time resources for the antidrug crime activities of the police were strongly increased.

In the research literature on drug control policy in Denmark, the term "drug institution" has been discussed (Laursen Storgaard 2000; Winsløw 1984). This concept is used to see the drug situation and the drug efforts as a context in which importance is given to the dynamics in a process wherein drugs as a social problem are becoming institutionalized. Social institutions are formed and reformed with recurring social activity. The repetition of control and management techniques, strategies, and behavior patterns by different actors is fundamental for the continuity of institutions (Giddens 1987). The development of Danish drug institutions would appear to confirm that the circulation of discourse and policy has created a foundation on which the institution has slowly begun to live as a self-generating system.

Starting with the concept of the drug institution, an attempt has been made to divide the development in the field since 1965 so as to define the qualitative changes in the development process. The years 1965 to 2000 have been divided into three so-called break periods and three so-called transition periods (Laursen Storgaard 2000). A break period is characterized by qualitative changes in the drug control policy as a result of more quantitative accumulation in the previous transition period. It is then possible to determine the following division into periods.

The first break period was determined to be the years 1968 to 1972, when the treatment and control systems were built up. By the end of the first break period in 1972, the Danish drug control system had been fundamentally changed from a control system relating to drugs prescribed under medical law to a penal law–oriented system to handle the new situation connected with young people's use of drugs, with its supply side connected to international drug crime. At this time, drug policy and the drug discourse basically concerned only cannabis. The principal discussion about control policy toward cannabis—that is, Should it be legalized, decriminalized, or handled from a restrictive attitude?—was the governing policy question in the drug discourse in the years 1968 to 1972. Although the prohibitionists won this discourse and in general managed to get control policy defined as restrictive, the cannabis liberalists succeeded in influencing regulation of prosecution and court practice in a lenient direction. A threefold rise of drug penalties in 1969 and the discussion about the consequences to the users led to the attorney general's circular in 1969 on prosecution practice, wherein it was pointed out that possession of small amounts of drugs for one's own use should be met with lenient measures, that is, warning for first-time appearance. In reality, this implied different policies on cannabis versus so-called hard drugs and on users versus dealers, which became a fundamental feature of Danish drug control policy.

The first transition period then follows as the years 1973 to 1978, when the drug abuse problem changed its character to become a persistent social problem and when the treatment of drug addiction was finally professionalized. The rest of the 1970s went to an end with only quantitative changes in the drug control system. In 1975, the maximum penalty was raised again, this time to imprisonment up to ten years in an attempt to meet the challenge from more and more professional drug criminals. According to penal code section 88, this can be supplemented with up to an extra five years in "particularly aggravating circumstances" wherein several offenses are being adjudicated at the same time.

The second break period can be located with the years 1979 to 1984. During this period, there was a comprehensive debate about the development of both the control system and the treatment system, which resulted in a consolidation of the control system and a starting process of change in the treatment system. Around 1980, two important factors began interplaying in the drug

institution. First, heroin began to dominate the drug market in the last half of the 1970s, which shaped the drug problem as a traditional social problem with a relatively large group of heavy drug users who lived under poor social and health conditions. Second, as a result of this, the number of drug-related deaths increased dramatically from 80 in 1978 to 165 in 1980 (Laursen Storgaard 2000, 108).

This provoked a new round of extensions of the control system, this time predominantly not in the form of change of legislation but by widening the scope of control, giving more resources to police control, and attempting to legalize certain untraditional investigation methods. The police strengthened their activity toward traffickers of illegal drugs in combination with more direct action toward users. All the way up through the 1980s, this increase in law enforcement was supported by a general control optimism among politicians and other actors and a belief that the dual supply and demand control could solve the drug problem.

The second transition period follows as the years 1985 to 1993, with a quantitative accumulation of crisis features in the drug policy and the drug situation. Contrary to the general expectation, the extended drug control did not solve the problem. It only produced more control damage, which became a central part of the drug control discourse at the end of the 1980s. In the beginning of the 1990s, the criticism against the results of police initiatives toward the supply of illegal drugs to the Danish drug market was so massive that police authorities turned to attaching more importance to drug demand-reducing strategies.

This leads to the third break period, from 1994 to the present, when political adjustments were again made on the basis of a general political drug debate.

This new strategy was implemented with the street-level actions of the police department in Copenhagen in the years 1989 to 1994 aimed at both a cleanup of the conditions in the affected areas and a general prevention and market dispersion. But this switch in strategy was also ineffective and was followed by the critical point at which the social problems in the inner-city areas in Copenhagen, caused by heavy drug use, should be met with treatment and social efforts rather than with police actions.

This was pushed forward by the discussion in connection with the government's white paper from 1994 (mentioned above), which put Danish drug policy back into an old track in which drug addicts should be treated and not policed. In return for this, the police in 1996 got the opportunity to pursue street dealers more aggressively.

DEVELOPMENTS IN THE
DANISH TREATMENT SYSTEM

The period since the emergence of the modern drug phenomenon in the mid-1960s shows a shifting set of views of treatment philosophy in the three dominant spheres: the social welfare field, the public health sector, and the correctional system. They have to some extent followed different courses but also changed positions as one or the other sector at any moment might have the interest of the public and the politicians.

In the late 1960s and most of the 1970s, the social-pedagogical sector was the one getting the most attention and taking the lead in the discourse of drug policy and treatment goals and methods. The leading actors—initially primarily in Copenhagen—were psychologists and others in contact with the Copenhagen Youth Clinic, which had developed methods for dealing with youthful deviance among the socially deprived in the city (Mentalhygiejnisk Forskningsinstitut 1974). The clinic also attracted a group of adherents among social workers, psychiatrists, and lawyers who advocated a liberal drug policy and counteracted tendencies toward repressive action. This group of treatment optimists with a social-psychological philosophy set the spirit of discourse until the late 1960s, when repressive views gained the upper hand along with a shift in the problem panorama from rather innocuous cannabis use among a growing and visible hippie community to a more traditional and increasingly solid abuse of opioids.

In 1969, new legislation was passed (see the Development of Danish Drug Control Policy section above) that laid the basis for tougher law enforcement. At the same time, the hawks of public opinion—a group of psychiatrists and a number of parents of new youthful drug addicts along with political activists and law enforcement personnel—took the upper hand in the public debate. The liberal view was maintained to some extent, however, in the legal distinction between hard and soft drugs in relation to law enforcement, and the social-pedagogical treatment institutions were allowed to continue for some time.

During this period, the public health system, that is, somatic hospitals and psychiatric wards, were puzzled and insecure in relation to the new drug phenomena. Nevertheless, a not negligible number of youthful drug users were treated in psychiatric hospitals. In some psychiatric hospitals, the staff experimented with environmental therapy on the therapeutic community line, but most took a traditional approach of individual treatment (Haastrup 1973; Haastrup and Jepsen 1981). The correctional system was the one that could not refuse to take care of the influx of drug abusers who entered the prisons. In the early seventies, a number of experiments were undertaken, and the principle of attenuation was the dominant management principle.

The idea of applying methadone on a larger scale was discussed in the early seventies but turned down by the social-psychological treatment ideologists—as well as by most of the professional audience—as a sign of surrender to the drugs. On the other hand, it turned out that the results of the social-pedagogical treatment institutions were not so positive that they could continue to draw the economic support necessary for maintaining this part of the welfare system.

During the second half of the seventies and the first half of the eighties, the experimental, optimistic,

social-psychological treatment ideology and its institutional representations gradually fell into disrepute with the communes that had to foot the bills. First Copenhagen then a number of smaller municipalities terminated the institutions they had created, and an increasing number of their clients were back in the streets. Although some experimentation on an outpatient basis continued to exist in the Copenhagen municipal system even after the partial dissolution of the Youth Clinic, the tides of treatment sought other ways.

The "solution" became a rapid growth in methadone maintenance treatment, first via the general practitioners (GPs) on an individual basis and later in the form of semiprivate methadone clinics. The National Board of Health for many years continued to support this measure, which was in 1986 legitimated by an expert group under the National Alcohol and Narcotics Board in a publication with the symbol-laden title *Meeting Man Where He Is*[1] (Alkohol- og Narkotikarådet 1984). The way was opened to large-scale methadone maintenance. The initiative for and the ownership of the problem, to some extent, had shifted from the social welfare sector to the public health sphere.

In the early 1980s, methadone maintenance had been started and expanded by a private GP in Copenhagen who took in increasing numbers of opioid addicts in methadone treatment. There was little or no therapy attached. The National Board of Health after some time became concerned by the growth of an illicit market in methadone that seemed to emanate from this practice, and the patients in the program were not interested in any other "cure." The result was that the right to prescribe methadone was taken away from the GP and turned over to a limited number of his GP colleagues. The results of these measures also failed to meet expectations. In 1983, Winsløw and Ege published a serious critique of the poor results of these measures. They ascribed part of the responsibility for this situation to the lack of social welfare follow-up on the part of the Copenhagen municipal services.

Nevertheless, methadone maintenance programs continued to grow during the following years, and the methadone seemed to have a sedative effect not only on the opioid addicts but also on the municipal services, as the costs were minimal since nothing or little was attached in the way of social welfare measures (Jepsen 1996b). During the late 1980s and the 1990s, the number of addicts in methadone maintenance grew from around 900 in 1985—out of an estimated number of 10,000 addicts—to around 2,100 in 1991 and 3,000 in 1994. It rose further after the change in 1996 (see below) out of an estimated number of 12,500 addicts in the late 1990s.

On the other hand, in the streets of Copenhagen, police in 1989 and 1990 invested heavily in cleaning up the drug subcultures near the Central Railway station, based on increasing demands from local residents, hotels, and other business interests (Jepsen 1996a).

But the police cells and the correctional services were not able to handle this increased influx of customers. So some Copenhagen policemen sent the arrestees off for treatment at an entrepreneurial private institution that swept them away and kept them locked up, later to present the bill to the Copenhagen municipal services. An alliance was forged between the policemen in the streets and the private institution as a practical solution to the abdication of treatment responsibility by the municipality of Copenhagen.

The efforts to clean up the streets, however, were accompanied by a deterioration in the situation of the Copenhagen addicts. As mentioned above, the early 1990s saw a sharp increase in the number of drug-related deaths, and although a part of the increase occurred outside Copenhagen, part of the responsibility for the increase was blamed on police harassment of the addicts in the streets.

In 1994, the worries about drug-related deaths, dissatisfaction with the methadone programs, and the lack of social welfare measures grew to become almost a scandal. In a TV documentary, *The Road to Hell*, several drug policy experts proclaimed the drug war lost and pointed to the Swiss heroin experiments and Dutch drug policy as alternatives to the failed Danish policy.

In 1994, however, the government published the white paper mentioned in the introduction, produced jointly by the Ministries of Health, Justice, and Social Welfare. The paper, which to a large extent carries the stamp of the Ministry of Health, was a disappointment to those who had expected a new course in drug policy. Rather, it was more of the same, maintaining the traditional emphasis on prohibition, law enforcement, preventive information, and treatment, with a trifle of harm reduction philosophy added.

In reality, the following period showed little change in the fields of prevention and law enforcement, but during the years 1995 to 2000, heavy investments were made in treatment (Socialministeriet 1998). Of these, the main investments fell in the sector of inpatient treatment institutions. The period became one of growing treatment optimism. A variety of treatment models were tried out and evaluated (Pedersen 1999, 2000). In addition to the Phoenix House model imported to Denmark via Norway, the models included gestalt therapy in a small institution, a number of institutions based on the Minnesota or twelve-step model, and a new experimental institution built on adaptations of the principles of the Italian Projetto Uomo (Project Man). The state funds and the municipal funds interacted, and the field became attractive to professionals as well as to more opportunistic entrepreneurs. In other words, the social welfare sector regained the initiative and set the agenda for an active and optimistic development in the treatment system.

Up until 1996, all GPs who wanted to could prescribe methadone, but in the public health sector, a revamping of the methadone treatment system was introduced in 1996 by transferring responsibility for methadone and other maintenance or substitution therapy from the GPs and the private methadone clinics to new public clinics to be run by the counties.

Only occasionally, the prescriptions could now be handled through the GPs, but as it turned out to be difficult for the counties to provide the necessary dispensing clinics, an increasing number of GPs—and some of the previous semiprivate methadone clinics—were allowed to continue prescribing. Whereas the GPs have always been rather liberal in their prescription practices, several complaints have been heard that the county clinics are too stingy in their prescription practices, often going below the recommended dose of 60 ml. per day, starting with minimum doses of 25 to 40 ml. and reaching 60 ml. as an absolute maximum. It also became a problem that some clinics reacted to nonconformity by withdrawing the prescription and sending the addict down to the bottom of the waiting line, with resumption of heavy use as a probable result. Still, from 1995, the number of addicts in methadone maintenance (five months or more) rose from around 2,700 to around 4,500 in 1999.

An important part of the philosophy behind the change was that the substitution of opioids by methadone should be accompanied by well-developed and coordinated social-psychological treatment and welfare measures. This has become the new point of criticism, however, as many counties and municipalities have proved themselves unable to coordinate their work across administrative and political boundaries. Likewise, the investment in treatment and welfare measures has been lagging, so in many cases, long waiting lists have been the result of the change in systems (Socialministeriet 1998; Pedersen 2001). Instead of attracting drug addicts into treatment, some systems have pushed them away through control-oriented, paternalistic, and rigid patterns of administration (Narkotikarådet 1997, 2000).

The most positive development, however, has taken place in the sphere of voluntary assistance and low-threshold facilities run by charitable organizations or by ex-users groups with support from the municipalities or from central funds. The ex-users have, in cooperation with local administrators and politicians, been able to build up informal places of retreat (Væresteder, i.e., places to be) without pressures to enter treatment and without requirements of abstention. The use of drugs is not allowed inside, so smoking and injecting must take place outside. In a few places, however, the users' representatives, who run the places, unofficially (and secretly) allow injection of drugs brought in from the outside in the toilets. But there are no official treatment and no substitution drugs available.

In general, the official public health sector, both at the clinics and at the central administrative level, has turned out to be more reluctant to innovation and change. The central administration has been opposed to innovations such as a heroin trial on the Swiss model as well as to injection rooms and low-threshold facilities. Also, the Ministry of Health has blocked such measures with reference to international obligations, in spite of public preferences for them and in spite of the examples of Holland, Germany, and Switzerland demonstrating the practicability and usefulness of such schemes.

The correctional system has, in a way, been more open to experimentation than has the public health system. In 1995, a project on treatment as an alternative to imprisonment was instituted, evaluated (Storgaard 1999a), and then made permanent in the form of conditional suspended sentences; release to a treatment institution to serve the rest of a prison sentence was practiced; special "contract wards" were created in some prisons (Storgaard 1998), allowing certain privileges in return for self-regulated abstinence; and an outside treatment institution working on the Minnesota model was allowed to practice its treatment model inside a maximum-security prison (Storgaard 1999b). Free access to needles and syringes in the prisons, as it is practiced outside, has the prison service been restrictive, primarily influenced by negative attitudes among the custodial staff.

Generally speaking, evaluation studies show that the result of inpatient treatment is an average retention rate after detoxification of 34 percent. After completion of treatment as planned, some 40 to 60 percent of this group are still drug free after one year (Pedersen 1999, 2000). The results of the treatment inside prisons or of the alternatives to prison are about the same (Storgaard 1999b).

The search for "the treatment" for drug addicts thus has reached a more realistic stage where expectations have been adjusted to more reasonable proportions. Still, for many, treatment works while it lasts. It thus becomes a question of how and at what cost this may be achieved. The Danish evaluation studies indicate some avenues for obtaining the best match between types of institutional treatment and types of clients. Thus, a person with a high score on intellectual openness has a greater likelihood of completing treatment of a psychotherapeutic, intellectualizing type, represented by two institutions in the study, where 63 percent completed the treatment as planned. However, persons scoring low on a five-factor checklist do not (the average rate of completion was 34 percent). They fare better in Minnesota-type institutions, where the former group does not (Pedersen 2000, 6).

The evaluation study recommends greater attention to placement, an increased use of systematization and knowledge, and an increased professionalization, not least in the inpatient institutions and in the referral organizations. Inpatient institutions in particular have been helping addicts achieve sustained abstinence from drugs after completion of the treatment program.

DISCUSSION

The history of the development in Danish drug policy as sketched here indicates that not one of the three (or four) pillars of policy can be said to have any preference over the others.

The repeated call for prevention—mostly in the form of calls for better information—has shown little effect in the face of youthful fashions and hard-core problems of abuse. The time for great campaigns against drug use—most recently the one against ecstasy—has passed, and skepticism prevails among professionals, while politicians continue to express their adherence to and belief in prevention and information (Teknologirådet 2001). It has been some comfort that surveys and qualitative studies indicate that the public scare about new designer drugs has grossly overestimated the extent of use of such drugs among the youthful clientele (Ribe Amt 2000; Frederiksberg Kommunes Rådgivnings Center 2001). But the fear of epidemics of cocaine and amphetamine use and of new synthetic drugs continues to linger and form the basis for repressive alerts.

Law enforcement, while heralded up until the mid-1990s, has lost much of its impetus and self-assuredness. More and more policemen, prosecutors, lawyers, and judges express their recognition of the limitations of this approach. None see it as a way to a solution of the drug problem or as a way to a drug-free society. Although seizures of large shipments of drugs either inside the country or outside, continue to be good media material, there is a growing recognition that only a small minority of the drugs are intercepted before they reach the national markets.

Police are also increasingly ambivalent about the impact of their street activities, although there remains widespread ritual adherence to the obligation to pursue law violators and even—among some—to confiscate drugs found on addicts. Other policemen, however, are ready to recommend legal drug supply of heroin to far-gone addicts and occasionally do so even in widely read newspapers—not to mention in private. There is thus a growing gap between the private problem definitions of actors and the official policy statements—and, in particular, between the quietly expressed skepticism of law enforcement officials and the continued unrealistic perception of the prospects of prohibition among right-wing politicians. Still, the rhetoric of prohibition continues to dominate official statements.

The treatment sector has had its ups and downs. Today, the heavy investments in the social and pedagogical sector form the basis for a steadily growing treatment system, and a growing number of professionals have begun to envisage the system as representing good career opportunities. There have been variations in the treatment philosophies of various schools including those that believe in abstention as a close, realistic, and all-dominant goal, particularly those adhering to the twelve-step model, and those that accept a wide variety of options, including substitution programs. The inertia of such systems, once established, will probably keep this sector alive and active during the coming years, although with a high rate of mortality among the more speculative types of institutions. Also, the expectations for outcomes have been adjusted to more realistic levels. And there is renewed room for experimentation in the outpatient field and for better coordination with the medical sector.

The public health sector, on the other hand, seems to be the most problematic. In practice, the public health approach has proven to be rather rigid, paternalistic, and opposed to change and experimentation. Although public health has an immediate ring of something positive, its actual practice and the way it is administered works to alienate the systems from the daily lives and needs of drug addicts (Narkotikarådet 2000).

In this situation, the way around the deadlock between social welfare and public health seems to go via the harm reduction development. Although this approach should be close to the ideology of public health and medical practice, the Danish public health system seems more attuned to regulation and control than to meeting the needs of drug abusers on a realistic, unprejudiced level.

It is ironic that in Denmark the development seems to indicate that the war on drugs is advanced as much by the central public health administration as by the law enforcement sector as a whole (Jepsen 2001).

In conclusion, therefore, the relevant parts of drug policy are to be found within the social welfare sector and the harm reduction approach, while the public health sector and the law enforcement sector continue to administer the prohibitionist approach from a philosophy of deterrence. The sectors of treatment and harm reduction have to fight these barriers to deliver as much of their badly needed services as possible.

Note

1. This is a quote from the Danish philosopher Soren Kierkegaard.

References

Alkohol- og Narkotikarådet. 1984. *At møde mennesket hvor det er* (Meeting man where he is). Copenhagen, Denmark: Alkohol- og Narkotikarådet.

European Monitoring Centre on Drugs and Drug Addiction (EMCDDA). 1999. *Udbredelse, forbrugsmønstre og konsekvenser af stofbrug* (Prevalence, patterns of use, and consequences of drug use). Lisbon, Portugal: European Monitoring Centre on Drugs and Drug Addiction.

Frederiksberg Kommunes Rådgivnings Center. 2001. *Ungdomsundersøgelsen 2000* (The year 2000 youth study). Frederiksberg, Denmark: Frederiksberg Kommune.

Giddens, A. 1987. *Social theory and modern sociology.* Cambridge, UK: Polity.

Haastrup, S. 1973. Young drug abusers: 350 patients interviewed at admission and followed up three years later. Ph.D. thesis, Munksgaard, Copenhagen.

Haastrup, S., and P. Jepsen. 1981. *350 patients followed up after 7 years.* Copenhagen, Denmark: Sundheds- og Socialforvaltningen.

Jepsen, J. 1996a. Copenhagen—A war on socially marginal people. In *European drug policy and law enforcement*, edited by N. Dorn, J. Jepsen, and E. Savona. London: Macmillan.

———. 1996b. Methadone as substitution for treatment? Recent developments in Danish methadone policy. In *Metadon—politik og etik. 4 konferenceoplæg. CRF-arbejdspapir*, 13-27. Aarhus, Denmark: Center for Rusmiddelforskning.

———. 2001. Narkotikakrigens Ofre (The victims of the war on drugs).

Working paper, University of Aarhus, Denmark, CRF.

Justitsministeriet, Socialministeriet og Sundhedsministeriet. 1994. *Bekæmpelse af narkotikamisbruget* (Fighting drug abuse—Governmental white paper). Copenhagen, Denmark: Justitsministeriet, Socialministeriet og Sundhedsministeriet.

Kouvonen, P., P. Rosenqvist, and A. Skretting, eds. 2001. *Bruk, misbruk, marknad och reaktioner. Narkotikasituationen i Norden 1995-2000.* NAD publication no. 41. Helsinki, Finland: Nordic Council for Alcohol and Drug Research.

Laursen, L. 1996. Scandinavia's tug of war on drugs. In *Discussing drugs and control policy*, NAD publication 31, edited by P. Hakkarainen, L. Laursen, and C. Tigerstedt. Helsinki, Finland: Nordic Council for Alcohol and Drug Research.

Laursen Storgaard, L. 2000. *Konstruktionen af dansk narkotikakontrolpolitik siden 1965* (The construction of Danish drug control policy since 1965). Copenhagen, Denmark: Jurist- og Økonomforbundets Forlag.

Mentalhygiejnisk forskningsinstitut. 1974. *Stofmisbrugere—frivillig behandling. Klienter, behandlingssystem og behandlingseffekt ved Ungdomsklinikken og Dag- og Døgncentret i København* (Drug abusers: Voluntary treatment. Clients, treatment system and treatment effects at the youth clinic and Dag- og Døgncenteret in Copenhagen). Copenhagen, Denmark: Mentalhygiejnisk Forlag.

Narkotikarådet. 1997. *Metadonarbejdsgruppens kommentarer til det hidtidige forløb af omlægningen af metadonbehandlingen* (Comments from the Working Group on Methadone on the reorganization of methadone treatment). Copenhagen, Denmark: Narkotikarådet.

————. 2000. *Substitutionsbehandling: Rapport fra Narkotikarådets substitutionsarbejdsgruppe* (Substitution treatment: Report from the Working Group on Substitution). Copenhagen, Denmark: Narkotikarådet.

Parliamentary Committees on Health and on Social Affairs. 1998. Parliamentary hearing on the possible legalization of cannabis. Unpublished.

Pedersen, Mads Uffe. 1999. *Stofmisbrugere efter døgnbehandling* (Drug abusers after inpatient treatment). Aarhus, Denmark: Center for Rusmiddelforskning.

————. 2000. *Stofmisbrugere før, under og efter døgnbehandling* (Drug abusers before, during, and after inpatient treatment—Summary report). Aarhus, Denmark: Center for Rusmiddelforskning.

————. 2001. *Substitutionsbehandling* (Substitution treatment). Aarhus, Denmark: Center for Rusmiddelforskning.

Ribe Amt. 2000. *Undersøgelse af rusmiddelbrug og -kendskab hos unge på ungdomsuddannelser* (A study of drug use and knowledge among youth in the youth education sector). Ribe: Ribe Amt.

Socialministeriet, Den Sociale Ankestyrelse. 1998. *Narkofølgegruppens Rapport om Udviklingen på stofmisbrugsområdet 1995-97* (Report of the parliamentary follow-up group on investments in the drug abuse field). Copenhagen, Denmark: Socialministeriet.

Storgaard, A. 1998. *"Kontrakten." i Ringe Statsfængsel* (The contract ward at Ringe State Prison). Aarhus, Denmark: Center for Rusmiddelforskning.

————. 1999a. *Behandling i stedet for fængselsstraf til nogle kriminelle stofmisbrugere* (Treatment instead of prison for some drug dependent offenders). Aarhus, Denmark: Center for Rusmiddelforskning.

————. 1999b. *Straf og misbrugsbehandling under samme tag* (Punishment and treatment under the same roof). Aarhus, Denmark: Center for Rusmiddelforskning.

Sundhedsministeriet. 2000. *Modelamtsoplæg* (Suggestions for model counties). Copenhagen, Denmark: Sundhedsministeriet.

Sundhedsstyrelsen. 2000. *Unges brug af illegale rusmidler—en kvalitativ undersøgelse* (A qualitative study of abuse of illegal intoxicants among youth). Copenhagen, Denmark: Sundhedsstyrelsen.

————. 2001a. *Alkohol- og Narkotikastatistik 2001* (Statistics on alcohol and drugs). Copenhagen, Denmark: Sundhedsstyrelsen.

————. 2001b. *Narkotikasituationen i Danmark 2000* (The drug situation in Denmark 2000). Copenhagen, Denmark: Sundhedsstyrelsen.

————. 2001c. *Notat om formodede Ecstasy-dødsfald* (Note on presumed ecstasy deaths). Copenhagen, Denmark: Sundhedsstyrelsen.

————. 2001d. *Unge og stoffer: Rapport fra Narkotika Seminar 2000* (Youth and drugs: Report from a seminar on narcotics 2000). Copenhagen, Denmark: Sundhedsstyrelsen.

Teknologirådet. 2001. Hearing on youth and drugs, 24 January, Christiansborg, Denmark. Available from www.tekno.dk.

Winsløw, J. 1984. *Narreskibet* (Ship of fools). Holte, Denmark: SocPol.

Winsløw, J., and P. Ege. 1983. *Metadon—og hvad så?* (Methadone—And then what?). Copenhagen, Denmark: Alkohol- og Narkotikarådet.

Policy Paradigms, Ideas, and Interests: The Case of the French Public Health Policy toward Drug Abuse

By HENRI BERGERON and PIERRE KOPP

ABSTRACT: The goal of this article is to analyze (1) how and why French public policy of care to drug users remained until 1995 a policy primarily curative, devoted only to proven drug addicts, directed toward abstinence, and mobilizing mainly the psychotherapeutic techniques inspired by the psychoanalytical paradigm, whereas the majority of the other European countries, answering to the brutal epidemic of AIDS, had, as of the middle of the eighties, started a palliative policy of risk reduction envisaging, among other measurements, the massive distribution of substitute products such as methadone and (2) how and why France brutally revised its positions, in the middle of the nineties, to adopt a policy of harm reduction and by doing this aligned itself, more or less, with the orientations followed by the other European countries. This analysis led the authors to test some of the political science approaches that stress the role of ideas in policy-making processes.

Henri Bergeron is a sociologist and researcher at the Centre de Sociologie des Organisations, Paris, and is a chargé de cours at University of Paris I—La Sorbonne. His work has centered on (licit or illicit) drug policies in Europe.

Pierre Kopp is an economist and professor at Panthéon-Sorbonne University (Paris I). He is working on the efficiency of public policy in the field of drugs.

NOTE: This article is a rewritten and extended version of two others articles: Bergeron (1999a) and Bergeron (2001). Some of its conclusions were presented at a conference organized by Rosemary Taylor at the Center for European Studies at Harvard University, 26-28 January 2001, titled "Re-Thinking Social Protection: Citizenship and Social Policy in the Global Age."

THE FRENCH PUBLIC HEALTH
POLICY TOWARD DRUG ABUSE:
A LONG-LASTING
EXCEPTION IN EUROPE

The French public health policy
toward drug use and drug addiction
is known to be very singular in
Europe: the choices made by French
experts, administrations, and governments to cope with drug consumption were specific to France up
to 1995.

Before explaining why French
public policy toward drug users was
so distinct from that of other European countries, we first want to discuss some concepts that helped us to
build our argument. We would like to
make clear that there are two ways of
understanding the expression "public health policy to cope with drug
consumption." Following Gusfield
(1981), there exist a causalist strategy for drug health policy and a
consequentialist one.

The first strategy (the causalist
one) supposes to carry out a policy
with a primary aim of providing care
for drug addiction: in this case, you
need to understand what are the possible causes of drug addiction and as
such to carry out programs that care
or try to care for addiction. Here
again, there are two major possible
aims for drug addiction treatment:
either (1) abstinence is a main aim,
and a set of different therapeutic
techniques are available, each of
which is based on a specific etiologi-
cal theory (paradigm)—(a) therapeutic communities based on behavioral
psychology; (b) methadone treatment
with progressive withdrawal; (c)
ambulatory treatments, such as
psychotherapies inspired by

different kinds of psychology such as
psychoanalysis, cognitive psychology,
behaviorism, and so forth—or (2)
abstinence is not the proper aim for
drug addiction treatment, because
drug addiction is regarded as essentially caused by biological (and more
and more neurobiological) deficiency.
Thus, in this perspective, drug
addicts should be provided with substitution drugs throughout their
lives, as for diabetics. All those curative treatments then typically concern individuals who have already
experienced drug addiction for a long
time, who do not feel at ease anymore
with it, and who desire to withdraw
from what they more and more consider to be a dangerous habit.

The second strategy for a public
health policy toward drug consumption is the one in which the chief aim
is not to provide care for drug addiction, properly speaking, but to take
action on the social and medical consequences of drug consumption. It is
obvious that drug consumption,
especially for heroin, is a risky practice. In this perspective, among other
measures (such as needle exchanges,
first line aid centers, etc.), methadone treatment could be an appropriate indication. According to many
experts and physicians, methadone
could not only reduce the progression
of the AIDS epidemic (even if this
point is still very controversial) but
also create the conditions for drug
users to seek help with their respective health and social situations. In
this perspective, methadone could be
provided to an addict who, for example, does not want to kick his or her
habit; who, for instance, has to be
hospitalized for a long time or who

needs to rest for a while; who needs social aid such as housing, a job, administrative registration, and so forth. In this respect, providing a heroin addict with methadone is more a palliative and preventive than a curative practice. This policy is called harm reduction policy. Of course, those two aims are complementary, but the hierarchy established between them within a public health policy has important consequences, as we will see later on.

What was the French situation in 1994? In 1994, French public policy was principally oriented toward a curative perspective. Its major aim was abstinence, and above all, there was by and large only one kind of therapy developed all over the territory: psychotherapy inspired by psychoanalysis. The two other major curative treatments (therapeutic communities and methadone treatment) were not present in the French health landscape. Moreover, a preventive and palliative harm reduction policy had never been carried out in France, and the international contrast with other European countries was, in this aspect, astonishing. Everywhere else in Europe, from the mid-1980s for Great Britain and Holland and at the very end of the 1980s for Germany, Switzerland, Spain, and in some respects, Italy, a harm reduction policy had been implemented mostly in reaction to the appearance of the AIDS epidemic.[1]

In fact, the shift in French policy occurred in 1995. Slowly, from 1992 on, a group of actors from different origins (hospital physicians concerned with AIDS, members of nongovernmental organizations concerned with social and medical first aid, some drug addicts, some experts, etc.) started to demonstrate against the French public policy's major aims and against the professionals who, up to this time, had been the legitimate experts for the government on drug problems. Given this background, the aim of this article is to answer two main questions: (1) How can we understand the singular French situation? How do we account for the fact that the aims of French public policy remained for so long on a curative perspective with abstinence as the ultimate goal? How can we understand that methadone had never been considered an acceptable and appropriate treatment by French experts whereas it was in almost all other European countries? Put differently, how do we explain the success of a policy (even by the standard of the French experts who were first against the development of methadone) that was not even recognized a few years earlier? and (2) How can we understand the disruptive shift that occurred within the French public policy toward a harm reduction policy?

THE STABILITY OF THE FRENCH PUBLIC POLICY

France has been characterized by a politics that led simple users to prison. Since 1998, things have been changing; both the number of sentences for drug use and the length of jail sentences are decreasing (see Table 1).

We can start our explanation of this singular situation by paying attention to institutional conditions.

TABLE 1
FRANCE DATA: 1999-2000

Number of problematic users	124,000-176,000
Number of substitution treatments	64,500
Number of arrests for consumption	74,633
Number of arrests for street resale	10,874
Sentences for drug use	70,444
Sentences for use and resale	6,530
Number of incarcerated people in the year	700

SOURCE: Observatoire Français des Drogues et des Toxicomanies (1999).

The French health tradition had always utilized, up to the late 1980s, a curative perspective when dealing with public health problems. This is a tradition in which prevention has long been regarded as a secondary aim. As a result, when the French state implemented a health policy toward drug users at the beginning of the 1970s, it did so to favor curative solutions. The French state was less inclined to carry out a preventive and palliative policy to which the recent introduction of methadone treatments is linked. But more fundamentally, we can also argue, to explain the French exception, that the majority of the critical actors and experts on this topic had slowly adopted a certain kind of paradigm to understand drug addiction. This paradigm was, among other references, largely influenced by psychoanalysis. This tradition's major arguments can be summarized as follows: taking actions to care for drug consumption consequences would entail more the implementation of a political will of social control than a therapeutic solution to drug addiction. (These experts, in the 1970s, were strongly influenced by Foucault's thesis, and many of them were very active in the "May 1968" revolution and/or in the French antipsychiatry movement.) Such a policy would have been, according to them, a policy that ignores the suffering "subject" who is hidden by a social stigma. On the contrary, by their logic, curing drug addiction, setting drug addicts free from their habit, would put them in better condition to get jobs, to find housing, and so forth: in one word, to recover a "normal" life since this rehabilitation would be grounded in a nonpsychopathological basis. Concerning methadone, they argued that since drug addiction is the symptom of deep psychological suffering, and since drug addiction is the symptom of psychopathological structures like neurosis, psychosis, or perversion, providing drug addicts with methadone would be providing them with simply another drug. With these two explanations in mind (the curative tradition and the domination of the psychoanalysis paradigm), it seems easy to see how a public policy that was principally curative emerged and for which methadone was morally (argument of social control) and scientifically (psychoanalytical arguments) unacceptable. But these explanations alone are not sufficient: we want to understand why and how the domination of a certain paradigm could have been possible in France.

Conceptualizing our issue in terms of a domination of a certain paradigm—interpretive framework—

(which involves certain aims, a certain hierarchy of those aims, certain instruments and solutions, specific settings of these instruments and solutions) led us to test the political science approaches that stress the role of ideas in policy-making processes.

Following Hall (1993),[2] we identify the groups of critical actors who succeeded in influencing the definition of what should and should not be French policy toward drug users. In other words, we tried to show how certain ideas became legitimate in the field and how some actors, taking advantage of their position on a "broader institutional framework" (Hall 1993, 280)—and convinced that the aims and solutions that derive from the psychoanalysis paradigm were the "right and proper things" to do at that time—succeeded in institutionalizing those ideas "into the standard operating procedures of key organizations and absorbed into the worldviews of those who manage them" (Hall 1997, 184). In this perspective, since the mid-1970s, a "policy network," formed by two major groups of actors, slowly took power in the field (Bergeron 1999b). As in many French public policy studies (see, e.g., Muller 1984, 1989; Setbon 1993), a policy network—in our case a policy community—gathered different kinds of actors sharing a set of common normative and cognitive ideas (involving certain aims, solutions, etc.), took advantage of the centralization of the French state (institutional conditions), and dominated the field. On one hand, a certain kind of professional—most of them psychiatrists—slowly eliminated

(during the 1970s) the competition of other experts who tried to promote other aims and solutions (therapeutic communities and methadone treatments) related to other paradigms and how they succeeded in being the legitimate representatives of the field for the French authorities (during the 1980s). On the other hand, a particular governmental agency (Direction Générale de la Santé, which is located in the French Health Ministry) also succeeded in appropriating the policy as far as financing, regulating, and evaluating the policy actions are concerned. Finally, these two groups of actors, civil servants, and professional experts obtained more and more autonomy in managing French public policy and how they struggled to keep actors, such as other agencies (namely, the Direction de l'Action Sociale of the French Health Ministry and the Mission interministérielle à la lutte contre la toxicomanie), other professionals, local authorities, and so forth away from involvement in French policy.

We should also mention that their actions and their monopolistic position in this field were possible because their aims and solutions were respected and were not in contradiction with the more global political and cultural norms (Bergeron 1998, 1999b). Ehrenberg (1993, 1995) showed very well that in France, drug addiction was clearly framed in terms of individual responsibility and that for this reason, most politicians would consider harm reduction policy as if they were "abandoning drug addicts to their addiction" and methadone as a "passive" instrument of getting out of addiction. With this fact in mind, there existed in France an objective alliance between politicians and psychiatrists inspired by psychoanalysis, who both, for different reasons, rejected consequentialist policy and methadone. But why did anomalous developments (the spread of AIDS and the degradation of the social conditions of many drug addicts) not threaten the French paradigm, whereas they had in other European countries, especially in those that had also implemented a mostly curative policy (Germany or Spain, for instance)?

We use Raymond Boudon (1986, 1990, 1995) who, inspired by Simmel and Weber, suggested taking into account the good reasons that actors have to believe in certain ideas and thus to act as they do (since a lot of actions are caused by beliefs). This perspective is rationalist in that it assumes that action is caused by reasons, whatever those reasons[3] could be: normative, cognitive, utilitarist, and so forth. Rationality[4] could then take the form of cost-benefit considerations in some circumstances but also other forms in other cases: the reasons an actor has to act as he does or to believe what he believes have to be perceived by the actor as strong and are not necessarily instrumental; the actor also endorses ideas because those ideas, to the best of his or her knowledge or normative dispositions, are acceptable. Endorsing a theory is in most cases an action caused by the fact that one sees strong reasons for endorsing it. In this respect, this approach shall not be reduced to the rational choice model, which, to put it briefly, considers individual actions to be essentially instrumental and mostly focuses on a certain kind of reason: personal interests.

To make those reasons comprehensible (in the sense of Weber, *verstehend*), we have to reconstruct the social, normative, and cognitive context in which the actors were situated before 1993. We have, in other words, to understand why certain ideas made sense for them at that time and in their social context. Here again, we shall be succinct: The reasons our experts and actors refused for so long to change French public policy on drugs and, especially, to introduce methadone treatments in France were influenced by two kinds of effects, called by Boudon (1986, 1990, 1995) "positional effect" and "dispositional effect."

The first one—positional effect—is a cognitive perspective. It basically supposes that you see reality according to the position you hold. Our hypothesis is thus: the experts and professionals who were working in therapeutic institutions and who were the legitimate advisors of French authorities concerning drug policy typically did not see, before 1993, drug addicts who presented the social and medical characteristics that convinced other European experts to reconsider their policy's aims and to adopt methadone treatment and harm reduction policies. In other words, they typically saw, during the 1980s and at the beginning of the 1990s, drug addicts who were not in such poor shape regarding health and social conditions. As a matter of fact, when in 1995-1996 methadone was finally provided to many French addicts, a population of addicts they had not previously encountered suddenly appeared in the treatment centers of those very experts. We cannot here explain why they confronted themselves with a certain kind of addict whose typical characteristics did not disturb their beliefs and were assumable by their paradigm, but we can suggest that it is linked to the way they were organized, the way they recruited patients, the therapeutic practices they used to care for patients, and so forth (Bergeron 1999b). Finally, consistent with the conclusion of the sociology of medicine (see, e.g., Freidson 1970) or of social aid organizations (see, e.g., Lipsky 1980), each field and organization tends to create and select its appropriate client, whose characteristics tend to confirm professional beliefs or at least not jeopardize them.

The second effect—dispositional effect—entails the process by which theories or systems of ideas to which one adheres slowly become a cognitive frame through which reality is interpreted in a specific direction. We can here give the example of a certain kind of drug addict who came in small numbers to the treatment centers during the 1980s and at the beginning of the 1990s could not end their heroin consumption with psychotherapy and underwent repeated detoxification treatments. Those patients are today regarded as one of the first targets for methadone treatment. But in those times, experts and professionals, according to their psychoanalytic point of view, would conclude that those addicts were not motivated enough to stop

addiction and to reconsider their past. They would conclude that a "free demand," as psychoanalysts tend to say, had not yet emerged and, therefore, were unsuited for methadone treatment. It is an obvious conclusion that actors tend (but not eternally) to select facts that confirm their beliefs. In this respect, the psychoanalytical paradigm slowly became an institution in the sense of Berger and Luckmann (1966). We can say, following Gusfield (1981), that methadone was at that time an "unthinkable" instrument for experts and civil servants. This fact also suggests that the accumulation of anomalies is not sufficient to threaten a paradigm, that ad hoc hypothesis, as Kuhn ([1962] 1970) showed, is often elaborated to cope with what is not yet perceived as an anomaly. It suggests then that change in ideas is a long-term process that requires several conditions to fully occur (see below).

Finally, policy making from 1970 to 1992-1993 was doubly autonomous: at the top since no contests and exogenous actors could interfere in the policy-making process (a "relatively closed policy network"; Hall 1993, 291) and at the bottom since the legitimate experts for the French government working in therapeutic centers were not in contact with a large part of the population of drug addicts and/or could not see anomalies as real anomalies.

But one must not insist too much solely on cognitive processes. Interest (personal utility) could also be a good reason to believe in certain ideas. That is why, inspired by the theory of organization that was promoted by

Crozier and Friedberg (1977), we added a third effect that we called "situational effect." The history we draw is also a story describing how a certain kind of professional took power in the field, how certain solutions, financing systems, typical ways of organizing activities were born; how ways of working, roles, practices, norms, hierarchies of personnel, professional identities, and so forth emerged and become institutionalized (Bergeron 1999b). Put simply, it is an account of how French public policy generated a special social world oriented by a particular scenario, a world confronting actors with a more or less stabilized system of power relationships. We should notice that by reconstructing this social world and the system of power relationships that goes with it, one may then be able to "capture dimensions of human interaction" (Hall 1997, 185) and then give an interactionist dimension to methodological individualism, which is often and wrongly accused of presenting an atomistic conception of actors. In fact, the history we draw is the story of how public policy concerning drug use and drug problems slowly became a public policy for drug addiction and even more for a certain kind of drug addict, that required certain kinds of expertise and experts. The major aims of the French public policy have slowly become more or less isomorphic to the aspirations of a certain type of professional (mainly psychiatrists believing in the psychoanalysis paradigm). It has become a social world in which many actors are embedded and linked to many different kinds of routines and interests, which would tend to strengthen their beliefs in certain ideas.

POLICY PARADIGM CHANGE

We use this approach to analyze the change in paradigm that shifted French policy from a curative policy dealing with the individual causes of drug addiction to a palliative and preventive one mostly focused on the social and medical consequences of drug consumption. As mentioned in the introduction, the shift in French policy occurred in 1995. Here again, we can follow Hall's (1993, 1997) model. Slowly, from 1992 on, a group of actors from different origins (hospital physicians concerned with AIDS, members of nongovernmental organizations, some drug addicts, some experts of the orthodox field that converted themselves to the harm reduction paradigm, etc.) started to demonstrate against the French public policy's major aims and against the professionals who, up to this time, had been the legitimate experts for the government on drug problems. For three years, a deep controversy raged, and this new policy network took advantage of a set of different conditions to change the hierarchy of goals guiding policy and the set of instruments employed.

The shift toward the harm reduction paradigm[5] took place as part of a more general change concerning the representation of what should be an appropriate public health policy at the beginning of the 1990s. The appearance of AIDS in Europe and in France revealed more accurately the failures of the curative tradition in public health policy, which led to terrible consequences for certain kinds of patients (what we call in France *le procès du sang contaminé* has been a traumatic event for French politicians). Those failures made preventive and palliative actions toward patients more legitimate aims in the French medical field. As a result, but later, in the specific field of drug policy, ideas stemming from the harm reduction paradigm, congruent with this more global transformation, slowly became more and more acceptable; such ideas became more "persuasive in themselves, which is to say, at least partially independently of the power of their proponents" (Hall 1997, 185). They had a cognitive and an axiological rationality in this new context. In this respect, an external group of different actors, helped by media that slowly became conduits for their ideas (the daily newspapers and TV), published a lot of reports on anomalous developments and, by doing so, made them visible in the public arena.[6] They presented the French situation as an exception in Europe; and succeeded in convincing politicians—above all the new government formed in 1993 by Edouard Balladur and especially Simone Veil, the freshly named minister of health— that methadone could be a means of stopping the propagation of AIDS and could create the conditions for drug users to seek help on their respective health and social situations.

We can conclude that French policy also "changed, not as a result of autonomous action by the state, but in response to an evolving societal debate that soon became" more or less[7] "bound up with electoral competition" (Hall 1993, 288). The new community policy, taking advantage of the *Sang contaminé* political trauma, succeeded in gaining authority in the field (the new visibility of anomalous developments contributed to undermining the authority of the orthodox experts and of the paradigm they advocated in favor of physicians dealing with AIDS in public hospitals). The development of methadone programs in France was then also (but not only) decided by Simone Veil on the argument that there exists a causal link between development of methadone programs and low prevalence of AIDS in the rest of Europe. But this causality was at that time very controversial and still is today. So to understand how new critical actors succeed in being regarded as authoritative for politicians, one must study not only the scientific debates in which experts in competition produce contradictory experimental proofs (causal link between AIDS prevalence and methadone programs) but also the links existing between the different competing paradigms and the more global institutional and cultural norms and values that also give selectively more legitimacy to certain scientific ideas and less to others. As Hall (1993) put it, one must notice that in this process, "shifts in the locus of authority" are very important:

Faced with conflicting opinions from the experts, politicians will have to decide whom to regard as authoritative, especially on matters of technical complexity, and the policy community will engage in a contest for authority over the issues at hand. In other words, the movement from one paradigm to another is likely to be preceded by significant shifts in the locus of authority over policy. (P. 280)

But once again, if you want to understand how "ideas can be persuasive in themselves" (Hall 1997, 185), the Boudon (1986, 1990, 1995) model seems necessary. It helps explain why, for instance, some of the experts of the orthodox paradigm converted to harm reduction before 1993 and then why they started to fight for the introduction of methadone in France. One can see that they were mostly located in a position in which they saw more anomalies (e.g., they were located in poor suburbs outside Paris and big cities) and that they tended to be less cognitively disposed to form ad hoc hypotheses when confronted with these anomalies. Endorsing the harm reduction paradigm was a rational action as far as cognitive and axiological rationalities are concerned. But these actors were also less interested in the social world institutionalized by the former policy. Thus, the reasons they switched to the harm reduction paradigm are clear: it served their personal utilities, of course, but it above all fit with their specific situation; helped them reconceptualize their past experiences through this new cognitive framework of anomalous experiences as real anomalies; offered a new professional identity;[8] helped them feel included in a larger community, backed by a coherent system of ideas that tended to reduce the psychological cost of being deviant; and so forth. Once again, the reasons they changed their ideas concerning how to cope with drug problems made sense for them in their given context

and were simultaneously cognitive, normative, and utilitarian ones. This perspective helps explain why almost the whole majority of professionals finally accepted, more or less, the necessity of implementing a harm reduction policy despite their earlier beliefs. At that time, anomalies were made visible for everybody (through the action of media, namely), and a new social world in which it was possible to invest was slowly emerging.

CONCLUSION

Finally, we think that adding such a sociological perspective to ideas-oriented approaches in political science presents two major advantages.

First, it opens the black box of socialization and gives clues to explain how institutionalization takes place. Culturalist perspectives generally assume the fact that widespread beliefs can be well explained by socialization processes: individuals involved in a certain kind of institutional environment are considered to interiorize norms, values, cognitive frames, beliefs, and so forth. To explain why beliefs spread in society, those kinds of perspectives mobilize the concept of interiorization. But labeling a process is not explaining the process. By reconstructing the different kinds of reasons an actor has to believe in certain ideas—ideas that are of course available in a certain social context and at a given time—and at the same moment explaining why those ideas make sense for him or her, you not only explain the phenomenological fact of conviction that actors express toward certain ideas but also open the black box of socialization, which in this respect turns out not to be so nebulous. Socialization describes the processes by which an idea can make sense, in many different ways, for an actor located in a particular cognitive, normative, and social context. Finally, interiorization (and cognitive frames that could result from this cognitive process) appears much more as a consequence of socialization than as its cause at the individual level.

Second, this approach offers the possibility of recognizing that beliefs and actions of individuals have to be viewed in multiple dimensions. In this perspective, it then appears obvious that the reasons actors have to believe in certain ideas and/or to act as they do could be cognitive, normative, and/or utilitarian ones (material interests, interests in terms of power, interests in terms of preserving a professional identity, interests in gaining legitimacy, etc.). Our study showed that at a certain period of the history of our policy, it was quite difficult for a sociologist to establish that beliefs of individuals determine their interests. We shed light on the fact that in our case, at a certain time, interests could be also (but not only) a good reason for believing and especially for continuing to believe in certain ideas. Finally, in such a perspective, ideas do not appear to be either rationalizations of self-interests or substantial entities, purely persuasive in themselves, endorsed by actors who would not be embedded in a social context.

Notes

1. As a matter of fact, you could, in February 1994, count up to 9,500 drug users provided with methadone treatment in Spain, 17,000 in Great Britain, 15,000 in Italy, 10,000 in Switzerland, and 8,000 in Holland. During the same period in France, only 77 drug users were provided with methadone, whereas the population of heroin users was estimated between 130,000 and 180,000 people. For three years, a deep controversy raged, at the end of which French authorities decided to develop methadone and other substitution treatments and to carry out a harm reduction policy. Today, there are as many as 70,000 drug users provided with substitution treatments in France.

2. We focus on Hall's (1993) theory and try to apply it to this different subject presenting an equal amount of "highly technical issues and a body of specialized knowledge pertaining to them" (p. 291).

3. Of course, those good reasons can lead to false beliefs. Those good reasons are then not "objective" reasons but reasons that make sense for the actor. True and false beliefs, according to Boudon (1986, 1990, 1995), should both be explained by this "cognitivist" approach.

4. Boudon (1986, 1990, 1995) rejected explanations that consider beliefs or actions caused not by reasons such as, for instance, the concept of habitus of Bourdieu (1980) or the "prelogical mentality" of Lévy-Bruhl ([1922] 1960).

5. There exists a huge literature constituting harm reduction—not as a paradigm but as a coherent system of normative and cognitive ideas.

6. A fascinating fact (which confirms the influence of our positional effect) is that during the "normal" period (1980s) and at the beginning of the public controversy in 1992, when TV reported on the dramatic social and medical situations of heroin addicts in Switzerland, for instance, where in the middle of big cities such as Zurich there are very special police-free places (they call them *scènes*) where addicts can get heroin and inject it, the orthodox experts tended to think that they in France succeeded in avoiding such misery.

7. As Hall (1993) observed, elections and formation of new governments are only one of

the different components that make change occur; before 1993, there had been other changes in government in France, which had little impact on the major goals of the policy.

8. Muller (2000) insisted on the fact that a change in *Référentiel* generally has heavy consequences on collective identities, consequences that explain partly the resistance to disruptive, normative, and cognitive changes.

References

Berger, P., and T. Luckmann. 1966. *The social construction of reality*. Garden City, NY: Doubleday.

Bergeron, H. 1998. Comment soigner les toxicomanes? *Sociétal* (June-July): 45-49.

———. 1999a. Croyances et changement: Le refus français de la méthadone. In *Les Drogues en France: Politiques, marchés, usages*, edited by C. Faugeron, 224-33. Geneva, Switzerland: Georg.

———. 1999b. *L'État et la toxicomanie: Histoire d'une singularité française*. Paris: P.U.F.

———. 2001. Définition des drogues et gestion des toxicomanies. In *Qu'est-ce qu'une drogue?* edited by H. S. Becker. Paris: Atlantica-Séguier.

Boudon, R. 1986. *L'idéologie ou l'origine des idées reçues*. Paris: Le Seuil.

———. 1990. *L'art de se persuader, des idées douteuses, fragiles ou fausses*. Paris: Fayard.

———. 1995. *Le juste et le vrai: Études sur l'objectivité des valeurs et de la connaissance*. Paris: Fayard.

Bourdieu P. 1980. *Le sens pratique*. Paris: Les Editions de Minuit.

Crozier, M., and E. Friedberg. 1977. *L'acteur et le système*. Paris: Le Seuil.

Ehrenberg, A. 1993. Remarques sur les drogues dans l'équation française. *Interventions* 42:12-18.

———. 1995. *L'individu incertain*. Paris: Calmann-Lévy.

Freidson, E. 1970. *Profession of medicine*. New York: Harper & Row.

Gusfield, J. R. 1981. *The culture of public problems: Drinking-driving and the symbolic order*. Chicago: University of Chicago Press.

Hall, P. 1993. Policy paradigms, social learning, and the state: The case of economic policymaking in Britain. *Comparative Politics* 25 (3): 275-96.

———. 1997. The role of interests, institutions, and ideas in the comparative political economy of the industrialized nations. In *Comparative politics*, edited by M. Lichbach and A. Zuckerman, 174-207. Cambridge, UK: Cambridge University Press.

Kuhn T. S. [1962] 1970. *The structure of scientific revolutions*. Chicago: University of Chicago Press.

Lévy-Bruhl, L. [1922] 1960. *La mentalité primitive*. Paris: PUF.

Lipsky, M. 1980. *Street-level bureaucracy dilemmas of the individual in public services*. New York: Russell Sage.

Muller, P. 1984. *Le technocrate et le paysan: Essai sur la politique française de modernisation de l'agriculture de 1945 à nos jours*. Paris: Editions Ouvrières.

———. 1989. *Airbus: L'ambition européenne. Logique d'Etat, logique de marché*. Paris: L'Harmattan.

———. 2000. L'analyse cognitive des politiques publiques: Vers une sociologie politique de l'action publique. *Revue française de sciences politiques* 50 (2): 189-207.

Setbon M. 1993. *Pouvoirs contre sida, De la transfusion sanguine au dépistage: décisions et pratiques en France, Grande-Bretagne et Suède*. Paris, Le Seuil.

Decriminalization of
Drug Use in Portugal:
The Development of a Policy

By MIRJAM VAN HET LOO, INEKE VAN BEUSEKOM, and JAMES P. KAHAN

ABSTRACT: Drug use is an increasing problem in Portugal. In response, following the advice of a select committee, the Portuguese government has recently issued a number of laws implementing a strong harm-reductionistic orientation. The flagship of these laws is the decriminalization of the use and possession for use of drugs. Use and possession for use are now only administrative offenses; no distinction is made between different types of drugs (hard vs. soft drugs) or whether consumption is private or in public. Although most people favor decriminalization in principle, doubts have been expressed about the way the law will be implemented because the law only sets a framework for those communities that wish to undertake such activities—it is an enabling law. This has led to a considerable lack of clarity and increases the risk of dissimilarity of implementation in different parts of the country. The future will show the effects.

Mirjam van het Loo holds a master's degree in public administration. After her graduation, she conducted research on communication between local governments and their citizens. She has been working for RAND Europe since 1996 in the areas of health care, drug policy, government organization, science and technology policy, and immigration. She conducted a number of studies in Portugal on drug demand reduction services, regionalization, and drug policy.

Ineke van Beusekom has a master's degree in public administration. During her studies, she focused on organization and management of health care organizations, in particular the management of change. Within RAND Europe, she works in the field of health and society. Her project topics range from the assessment of the appropriateness of medical treatments to inventing ways to implement a country's national drug strategy.

James P. Kahan is the research director at RAND Europe. He has a Ph.D. in mathematical social psychology and a background in individual and small-group decision making. With RAND for more than twenty years, he has worked in every unit, on a wide variety of substantive topics. In recent years, Kahan has conducted a number of studies on regional development in Portugal and on drug policy.

49

P ORTUGAL began a remarkable experiment on 1 July 2001. It decriminalized all drugs, including heroin and cocaine, as well as marijuana. By decriminalization, we mean that use and possession for use are subject to administrative sanctions instead of criminal proceedings; in keeping with international treaties and the practice in other countries, Portugal is not prepared to legalize drugs. The decriminalization policy is the flagship of a revolutionary change in Portuguese drug policy, one of a number of harm reduction measures.

This revolutionary step began with the formation of an elite expert commission to consider what was widely regarded as an increasing drug use problem. The Commission for a National Drug Strategy (CNDS) produced a report (Comissão para a Estratégia Nacional de Combate à Droga 1998) recommending a major shift in Portuguese drug policy in the direction of harm reduction, including decriminalization. This shift was the logical development of an explicit set of basic principles for policy developed by the commission and did not consider the experiences of Spain or other countries (members of the CNDS, personal communications, March 1998 through November 2001).

To the surprise of some of the members of the CNDS, the Council of Ministers approved the report almost in its entirety (Government of Portugal 1999) and produced a national drug strategy consistent with that report (Government of Portugal 2000). The Assembleia da República (parliament) and Council of Ministers, with the approval of the president of the republic, passed specific implementation legislation, of which the most significant is the decriminalization law that took effect in July 2001.

In this article, we shall provide some background information on drugs and drug usage in Portugal and trace the development of the changes in Portuguese drug policy and what the anticipated results of the changes will be. Because this is policy in the making, with changes sometimes occurring on a daily basis, our description is largely based on a series of interviews and discussions dating from March 1998 through July 2001, conducted in Portugal, with more than thirty-five people involved in this process. The interviewees were, among others, most of the members of the CNDS, members of parliament, a Supreme Court justice, the mayor of Lisboa, members of treatment delivery organizations from different parts of the country, and the leadership of the Institute for Drugs and Drug Addiction (Instituto Português da Droga e da Toxicodependência [IPDT]) and the Drug Prevention and Treatment Service (Serviço de Prevenção e Tratamento da Toxicodependência [SPTT]). These interviews have been

NOTE: Correspondence should be addressed to J. P. Kahan, RAND Europe, Newtonweg 1, 2333 CP Leiden, the Netherlands; e-mail: kahan@rand.org. We wish to thank the Association for Innovative Cooperation in Europe, the Luso-American Foundation for Development. We are grateful for a RAND President's Award for supporting the work behind and writing of this article.

reinforced by examining what data exist on the drug problem in Portugal and official governmental documents.

Setting the stage

Before we turn to drug policy in Portugal, we will provide some background information about the country itself. Modern Portugal has approximately 10 million inhabitants and has a total land area of about 92,000 square kilometers. The country occupies the western edge of the Iberian peninsula (except for Galician Spain in the northwest corner), plus the two island groups of the Azores and Madeira. Portugal is an old country, with borders pretty much the same for more than nine hundred years; it remains remarkably homogeneous in its culture, language, religion, and ethnicity. The twentieth century saw more than fifty-five years of dictatorship and poverty, ending with a bloodless revolution in 1974, which was followed by the establishment of solid democratic structures and the beginning of a remarkable period of economic growth. In 1986, Portugal entered the European Union (EU), and although still one of the poorer countries in the EU, it was one of the original eleven countries to join the euro zone in 1999. Perhaps in reaction to the years of dictatorship, current Portuguese political philosophy favors providing a strong degree of both individual liberty and autonomy to subnational government (Kahan et al. 1999); the latter is especially true for social services such as health, education, and the prevention and treatment of drug use.

PORTUGAL'S DRUG PROBLEM

The revolution of 1974 and economic growth of the past twenty-eight years have not been an unmixed blessing. With the transformation from a highly dispersed rural demography to concentration in cities—notably Lisboa and Porto—came some of the ills of modern society, including drug abuse. However, although there is widespread belief that Portugal's drug problem worsened in the 1990s, real data on the extent of the problem have remained scarce. Indeed, one of the first calls in the national drug strategy is for the collection of more reliable, valid, and comprehensive data on the drug phenomenon.

Data on drug usage and treatment

Although recent data suggest a population as high as 100,000 drug addicts, more usual and conservative estimates put the number of Portuguese drug users between 50,000 and 60,000 out of a total population of approximately 10 million people (www.drugtext.org/count/portugal/portugal1.html). One-third of both the general population and the population of drug users are concentrated in the Lisboa area.

Portuguese data on drug usage are scant and not reliable. There is no equivalent to the national surveys on drug use that take place in a number of North American and European countries. No data exist on the lifetime or last-twelve-months prevalence of drug use among the general population in Portugal. What data are collected are reported to the European Monitoring Center on Drugs and Drug Addiction (EMCDDA), which was set up (coincidentally, in Lisboa) to provide the European Commission and its member states with objective, reliable, and comparable information concerning drugs and drug addiction and their consequences and to collect information on drug use in each of the EU member states. The information below is available through EMCDDA (www.emcdda.org; EMCDDA 2001).

The data in Table 1, which experts claim stretch credulity, clearly indicate that the drug problem increased significantly during the 1990s.

The information depicted in Figure 1 places Portugal unfavorably with respect to other harm-reductionist countries, with thirty-four drug-related acute deaths per million citizens compared to four per million in the Netherlands, eight per million in Spain, and nineteen per million in Italy.

Data on criminal justice system activity with regard to drugs

Arrests for drug offenses reflect the increasing use of heroin. In 1991, 4,667 people were arrested for drug offenses. By 1995, this number was up to 6,380, and by 1998, the figure was 11,395 or 235 percent of the 1990 figure. In 1998, 61 percent of the arrests were for use or possession for use (as opposed to sale or possession for sale), and 45 percent of the arrests were heroin related. Given the overwhelming prominence of heroin in

drug treatment, these numbers are relatively low.

Table 2 provides information on seizures of drugs. This table is another indication that the heroin problem increased in the 1990s but that seizures of other drugs did not reflect the pattern of heroin. The quantities of ecstasy and LSD are so small that they cannot be used to

TABLE 1
STATISTICAL DESCRIPTION OF DRUG USE IN PORTUGAL

Lifetime prevalence of use of different illegal drugs among fifteen- to sixteen-year-old students (from a sample of 4,767 students, 1995) (%)	
All illegal drugs	4.7
Cannabis	3.8
LSD	0.2
Cocaine	1.0
Heroin	0.9
Characteristic of the persons treated for drug problems	
Mean age (years)	28.6
Gender = male (%)	84
Heroin as main drug (%)	> 90
Injection as main route of administration (%)	42
Incidence of drug-related AIDS cases (annual incidence rates per million population)	
1985	0.1
1990	4.3
1995	39.5
1998	54.7
Prevalence of hepatitis C among drug injectors	
Lisboa, 252 people tested 1998-1999 (%)	74
Prevalence of HIV infection among drug injectors (%)	
Nationwide, 632 people tested 1998-1999	14
Lisboa sample	48

FIGURE 1
NUMBER OF ACUTE DRUG-RELATED DEATHS, 1987-1998

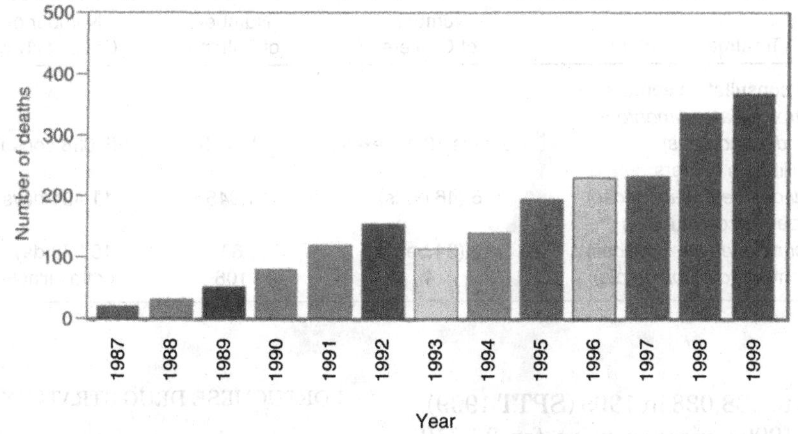

form reliable indicators of the extent of usage of these drugs.

Comparing Portugal to its neighboring countries, the number of heroin seizures per million inhabitants is quite low. Whereas the Portuguese police seize heroin 37 times per 1 million inhabitants, this number is 52 for the Netherlands, 337 for Spain, and 112 for Italy. It is inadvisable, however, to draw any conclusions about the heroin market in a country on the basis of these numbers because the number of seizures depends on a variety of factors, one of which is the effectiveness of the police. Still, one might expect Portuguese seizures to be higher given that its coastal access and links to Brazil make it an attractive transshipment country.

Treatment of drug addicts

The number of treatment episodes in Portugal has increased fivefold in the past nine years, from 56,438 in

TABLE 2
NUMBERS OF SEIZURES AND QUANTITIES OF DRUGS SEIZED IN PORTUGAL, 1990, 1995, AND 1998

Drug/Year	Number of Seizures per Year	Total Quantity per Year
Cannabis		
1990	1,279	9,606 kgs.
1995	914	7,493 kgs.
1998	2,063	5,582 kgs.
Heroin		
1990	1,346	36 kgs.
1995	2,828	66 kgs.
1998	3,750	97 kgs.
Cocaine		
1990	346	360 kgs.
1995	872	2,116 kgs.
1998	1,377	625 kgs.
Amphetamines		
1990	2	not available
1995	not available	not available
1998	1	not available
Ecstasy		
1990	not available	not available
1995	5	77 tablets
1998	35	1,127 tablets
LSD		
1990	not available	not available
1995	not available	11 doses
1998	10	261 doses

TABLE 3
TREATMENT IN PORTUGAL IN 1999, BY TYPE OF TREATMENT CENTER

Type of Treatment Center	Number of Centers	Number of Patients	Number of Consults/Days
Addict consultation centers (*centros de atendimento a toxicodependentes*)	40 (plus 10 annexes)	27,750	288,038 consults
Rehabilitation centers (*unidades de desabituacão*)	5 (46 beds)	1,945	11,431 days
Therapeutic communities (*comunidades terapeuticas*)	2 (34 beds)	63	10,578 days
Day centers (*centros de dia*)	4	106	not available

1990 to 288,038 in 1999 (SPTT 1999). The 1999 episodes were for 27,750 individual drug users, for an average of about 10.4 annual visits per user (see Table 3). Of all drug addicts undergoing treatment at treatment centers (*centros de atendimento a toxicodependentes*) in 1997, 95.4 percent were heroin users. Methadone, or LAAM, is not extensively used, being prescribed to only 21.8 percent of individuals in treatment. Treatment professionals in Portugal were long reluctant to treat heroin users in substitution programs because they did not believe in their effectiveness.

At a more operational level, the IPDT (a new organization begun in 2000) is responsible for the coordination of treatment and prevention. At the local level, it has district delegations, which allow closer proximity to the problems and the individuals. IPDT works in cooperation with ministerial services, such as the SPTT and the prevention programs in schools set up by the Ministry of Education (EMCDDA 2001) (see Figure 2).

PORTUGUESE DRUG STRATEGY

The CNDS was formed in response to a rapidly rising drug problem in the 1990s, principally but not exclusively involving heroin use. The path begun by CNDS and followed by the government makes clear that Portugal does not wish its policies to place it outside the mainstream of international drug policy. But Portugal is determined to implement a coherent and comprehensive strategy based on the philosophy of harm reduction, in the broad sense of referring to activities that reduce harm to the drug-consuming individual and society (see Table 4). In this broad sense of the term, all activities that reduce supply and demand and all activities that improve the situation of consumers can be considered harm reduction measures, including effective treatment and prevention (members of the CNDS, personal communica-tions, March 1998 through November 2001).

More information comes from eight structuring principles on which the strategy is built (Government of Portugal 2000, 39):

FIGURE 2
ORGANIZATIONAL CHART OF THE INSTITUTIONAL FRAMEWORK IN PORTUGAL

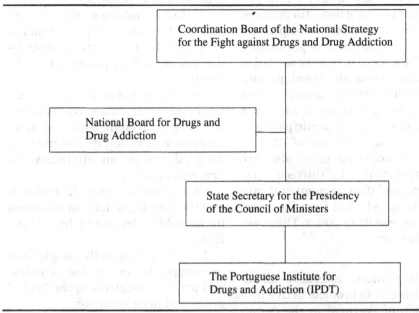

TABLE 4
GOVERNMENT BUDGET ON DRUGS AND DRUG ABUSE, BY INTERVENTION AREAS

1. the principle of international cooperation,
2. the principle of prevention,
3. the humanistic principle,
4. the principle of pragmatism,
5. the principle of security,
6. the principle of coordination and rationalization of resources,
7. the principle of subsidiarity, and
8. the principle of participation.

Intervention Area	Year 2000 Euro	Percentage
Prevention	24,150,976	23.3
Treatment	29,288,115	28.2
Rehabilitation	15,234,195	14.7
Harm reduction	4,589,728	4.4
Prisons	3,427,404	3.3
Law enforcement	24,007,142	23.2
Research	2,097,445	2.0
International cooperation	887,860	0.9
Total	103,682,864	100.0

SOURCE: Instituto Português da Droga e da Toxicodependência (2000).

These begin with acknowledgment of the international arena and acknowledge the importance of prevention, but then go immediately to the heart of the matter—the humanistic and pragmatic principles. These two declare that drug users are to be regarded as full members of society instead of cast out as criminals or other pariahs and that the strategy will not attempt to strive toward an unachievable perfection such as zero drug use but will instead try to make things better for all segments of society. The principle of security refers not only to the general public, as potential victims of drug-induced crime, but the drug users themselves. The remaining three principles reflect Portuguese political philosophy, with efficiency of resources needed to maintain economic development, subsidiarity part of a concerted effort to push policy making to as local a level as possible, and participation in a legacy of the revolution of 1974.

The structuring principles are translated into a set of thirteen "strategic options" (Government of Portugal 2000, 43-44) that form the heart of Portuguese drug policy. These are the following:

1. to reinforce international cooperation and to promote active participation of Portugal in the definition and evaluation of the strategies and policies of the international community and the EU;

2. to decriminalize the use of drugs, prohibiting them as a breach of administrative regulations;

3. to redirect the focus to primary prevention;

4. to extend and improve the quality and response capacity of the health care network for drug addicts, so as to ensure access to treatment for all drug addicts who seek treatment;

5. to extend harm reduction policies, namely, through syringe and needle exchange programs and the low-threshold administration of substitution drugs as well as the establishment of special information and motivation centers;

6. to promote and encourage the implementation of initiatives to support social and professional reintegration of drug addicts;

7. to guarantee conditions for access to treatment for imprisoned drug addicts and to extend harm reduction policies to prison establishments;

8. to guarantee the necessary mechanisms to allow the enforcement by competent bodies of measures such as voluntary treatment of drug addicts as an alternative to prison sentences;

9. to increase scientific research and the training of human resources in the field of drugs and drug addiction;

10. to establish methodologies and procedures for evaluation of public and private initiatives in the field of drugs and drug addiction;

11. to adopt a simplified model of interdepartmental political coordination for the development of the national drug strategy (IPDT replaces Projecto Vida);

12. to reinforce the combat against drug trafficking and money laundering and to improve the articulation between the different national and international authorities; and

13. to double public investment to 160 million euros (at the rhythm of 10 percent a year) during the next five years, so as to finance the implementation of the national drug strategy.

The first strategic option acknowledges the international context, but the second moves immediately to decriminalize the use of all drugs. Decriminalization, as is made clear, is not legalization but removal of sanctions for drug use from the criminal justice system.

Legislation

The thirteen strategic options have formed the basis for legislation and action plans that aim to set the legal framework for the strategy and its detailed implementation in a first stage between 2001 and 2004. During the past several months, laws and action plans have been issued for prevention, decriminalization, harm reduction, reintegration, and the combat against drug trafficking and money laundering. Furthermore, treatment capacity has increased to be able to respond to the expected increase of treatment demand as a consequence of the decriminalization law.

Prevention activities are to focus on primary prevention, in schools, families, and the community in general. Harm reduction measures (in the narrow sense of the term) include needle and syringe exchange, shooting rooms, information and motivation centers, and substitution programs. Decriminalization, as the flagship of the strategy in terms of its attention in the public eye and the complexity of its implementation, will be described here in greater detail.

DECRIMINALIZATION
OF DRUG POSSESSION

Decriminalization represents a significant departure from the previous law and is different from efforts in other countries such as Italy and Spain in that it explicitly separates the drug user from the criminal justice system. The CNDS recognized, and the government explicitly concurred, that imprisonment or fines have so far not provided an adequate response to the problem of mere drug use and that it has not been demonstrated that subjecting a user to criminal proceedings constitutes the most appropriate and effective means of intervention.

The international arena was explicitly addressed in deciding to adopt decriminalization. The national strategy document declared that after a study of the 1988 United Nations convention against illicit trafficking in narcotic drugs and psychotropic substances, it was consistent with that convention to adopt the strategic option of decriminalizing drug use as well as the possession and purchase for this use. In the Portuguese view, replacement of criminalization with mere breach of administrative regulations maintained the international obligation to establish in domestic law a prohibition of those activities and behaviors. Moreover, decriminalization as defined by the national strategy was the only alternative to maintaining drug use as a criminal offense that is compatible with the international conventions currently in effect (Government of Portugal 1999, 61).

How decriminalization will work

Under the law passed in October 2000 (Assembleia da República 2000) that took effect on 1 July 2001, the use and possession for use of drugs is no longer a criminal offense but instead is prohibited as an administrative offense. This distinguishes Portugal from Spain, where the policy is de facto decriminalization but where a drug consumer will still be judged by a criminal court, although he or she will never be sent to prison for drug consumption alone. The same holds for the American system of drug courts, which sends a drug consumer to treatment only after he has been convicted by a criminal court. Both in Spain and in the U.S. drug court system, the consumer has a criminal record, and it is this stigmatization that the Portuguese policy explicitly aims to prevent. There is no distinction made between different types of drugs (hard vs. soft drugs) or whether drug use is private or in public. Decriminalization refers only to possession of drugs for personal use and not for drug trafficking. "Trafficking" for purposes of the law is possession of more than the average dose for ten days of use (although what these levels are for specific drugs is not spelled out in the law).

To deal with these administrative offenses, each of the eighteen administrative districts in Portugal will establish at least one committee that deals only with drug use in that district (larger districts such as the ones containing Lisboa and Porto will probably have more than one committee). The committees will generally consist of three people, two people from the medical sector (physicians, psychologists, psychiatrists, or social workers) and one person with a legal background. Committee members are not supposed to be involved in drug treatment but should be sufficiently knowledgeable to judge what is best for the user.

Largely, drug users will be brought to the attention of the administrative committees when the police observe them using drugs. Although police will cite users and send the citation to the administrative committee, they will not arrest users. If the committee determines on the basis of the evidence brought before it that the person is a drug trafficker, then the committee will refer that person to the courts. Although the law states that any doctor who detects a drug problem in a patient may bring this to the attention of the committee in his or her district, it is regarded as highly unlikely; not only is such reporting repugnant to most doctors, but it might violate the doctor's oath of confidentiality.

The law states that the committee should consider a number of criteria in determining what action to take with a drug user. These criteria include the severity of the offense, the type of drug used, and whether use is in public or private; if the person is not an addict, whether use is occasional or habitual; and the personal and economic/financial circumstances of the user.

How these criteria are to be used is not stated. Some are of the opinion that the committee may choose not to take any action; others believe that some form of action, even if suspended, is required.

The committees have a broad range of sanctions available to them. These include the following:

- fines, ranging from 25 to 150 euros (these figures are based on the Portuguese minimum wage of about 330 euros [Banco de Portugal 2001] and translate into hours of work lost);
- suspension of the right to practice if the user has a licensed profession (e.g., medical doctor, taxi driver) and may endanger another person or someone's possessions;
- ban on visiting certain places (e.g., specific discotheques);
- ban on associating with specific other persons;
- interdiction to travel abroad;
- requirement to report periodically to the committee;
- withdrawal of the right to carry a gun;
- confiscation of personal possessions; and
- cessation of subsidies or allowances that a person receives from a public agency.

The committee cannot mandate compulsory treatment, although its orientation is to induce addicts to enter and remain in treatment. The committee has the explicit power to suspend sanctions conditional on voluntary entry into treatment, but because disobedience of committee rulings is not defined as a criminal offense, it is not clear what the further sanctions are if users do not follow either the treatment recommendations or the orders of the committee. Some experts believe that the committees will see users repeatedly and should build up a rela-tionship of trust with the addict. Other experts hold that this is not possible because the committee is acting as a judge and jury.

Preparations for decriminalization

IPDT is charged with overseeing the administrative committees (IPDT 2000). Since the passage of the law, it has been busy preparing for this. A major task is appointing committee members; IPDT organized a competition (*concours*) to select the members of the committees and their technical staff, and the committees were all in place on 1 July 2001. It is also attempting to specify a number of articles that were left vague in the law. Furthermore, IPDT has organized a training program for committee members, as well as a set of regulations for procedural matters and guidelines for how the committees should deal with cases. In addition to the administrative district committees, it will create a central committee that will serve as a center of information and advice to the districts.

IPDT has also begun designing a database in which information about the individuals brought before the committees, the decisions of the committees, and—to a more limited extent—the consequences of committee actions are recorded. They hope that this database can be employed to assist in standardizing the approaches of the committees and may, eventually, assist in evaluating the performance of the committees. Ultimately, the database plus the documented experience of the committees may assist in evaluating the effect of the strategy to decriminalize and in improving the law.

Beliefs about the likely effects of drug decriminalization

As decriminalization has barely begun, its effects cannot yet be measured. Plans are under way for major reforms in the collection and analysis of information about the number of drug users in Portugal, the extent of their use, and the consequences of such use on the users and others. In its most recent action plan, the government mentions its plan to conduct a major evaluation of the policy after a few years, although it is not yet clear who should conduct this evaluation and what it should focus on (Conselho de Ministros 2000). Among the people interviewed on this topic, there was a guarded optimism about the results of decriminalization and some consensus as to its anticipated consequences. These expectations can be used to form benchmarks for the evaluations. Almost all observers agree that evaluation is a useful tool for assessing the effectiveness of a policy, but there is a concern that the results of this particular evaluation would be subject to politically colored interpretations.

Decriminalization is not expected to increase the amount of drugs available or the use of new types of drugs. However, there is a general belief that decriminalization increases the need for prevention, for example, to communicate to the public that decriminalization does not condone drug use. The national drug strategy calls for increased prevention activities apart from decriminalization, but the effects of these two strategies are viewed as interdependent.

The Portuguese do not generally believe that decriminalization will result in an increase in the total number of drug users. However, there might be some increase in experimentation among those people who are deterred by fear of criminal sanctions. There is a consensus that decriminalization, by destigmatizing drug use, will bring a higher proportion of users into treatment, thereby increasing the need for treatment.

One could imagine that a final potential problem is that decriminalization may come to dominate the entire drug policy arena, with a corresponding diminution of important efforts in prevention, rehabilitation, and other programs consistent with the principles of humanism and pragmatism. On the other hand, one could also believe that decriminalization can act as a flagship for implementation of policies consistent with the structural principles and can ease the way for improved harm reduction strategies such as the introduction of new needle exchange programs, social housing for drug addicts, shooting rooms, more frequent supply of methadone, and consideration of heroin as a substitution drug. As this experiment unfolds, it will be interesting to see which direction it takes.

Other harm reduction activities

The Council of Ministers has recently published its action plan for the coming years, which includes prevention activities, experiments with shooting rooms, more treatment possibilities, and other implementations of the strategic options (Conselho de Ministros 2000). One experiment that has been in progress for a number of years now is the Casal Ventoso project. Casal Ventoso is a neighborhood of Lisboa where drug traffickers and drug users used to gather, to the detriment of themselves and the local inhabitants. The municipality of Lisboa has started a project wherein addicts are offered a place to wash, eat, and sleep; where clean needles are handed out; and where people get informed about treatment possibilities. This approach has proven successful because fewer people sleep in the streets and more addicts are induced to enter treatment or at least to inject hygienically.

Perceived problems
with implementation

Although most people favor decriminalization in principle, there have been a number of doubts expressed about the way the law will be implemented and, ultimately, its effects. The new law may be characterized as leaving unsaid more than it says. This has led to a considerable lack of clarity among the people who will be charged with implementing the law and those people who will be affected by the law. The committees will have to coordinate with each other and with people from other organizations, such as prevention workers and police. This is viewed as problematic, as there is no culture of coordination in Portugal, especially with regard to drug treatment (van het Loo et al. 2000).

There is confusion about the types of sanctions that could be given. Most people are aware of the range of possibilities mentioned in the law but do not see what criteria will be used by the committees to exercise which sanctions. The charge to the committees, to decide on the most appropriate sanction for the drug user, begs the question in absence of information about the effects of the sanctions. In principle, possession of all types of drugs is decriminalized. However, as explicitly mentioned as a possibility in the law, the types of sanctions prescribed by the committees might differ by type of drug used.

Some experts claim that the drug decriminalization law is a mere confirmation of current practice. Previously, these experts state, an addict would rarely be sent to prison for drug use alone, especially when the drug was cannabis; the police would arrest a person only if he or she were caught in another illegal action (e.g., stealing money) in addition to using drugs. Others do not see police behavior in this way and view the new law as an opportunity to reduce variation in practice in the direction of not labeling drug users as criminals.

There will probably be more people who apply for treatment since that is an escape from administrative sanctions. Many in SPTT and elsewhere believe that the current financial and human resources for treatment may not be adequate to receive this influx of new patients and worry that waiting lists from the committee referrals could become a major problem. There is also some concern about whether the modes of treatment currently used in Portugal are the right ones to meet the anticipated need for treatment. Some treatment specialists believe that more low-threshold methadone maintenance treatment is needed for the anticipated new population that will be seen.

There is some concern that the public does not (yet) understand what decriminalization is and confuses it with liberalization or legalization, thus sending a signal to the public that using drugs is not so bad after all. IPDT plans a public information campaign about the new law.

From an outsider's perspective, the administrative committees most resemble drug courts, as used in the United States and United Kingdom (Sechrest and Shicor 2001). However, neither IPDT nor any other organization in Portugal has to date shown awareness of the promises and pitfalls of drug courts, and there is a risk, sometimes explicitly expressed in Portugal, that the administrative committees will not be clearly differentiable from the current court procedures by users or the police. A particularly pessimistic view is that the committees are doomed to fail because of bad coordination and that the committees in fact mean that one police system is replaced by another police system.

The action plans regarding prevention, harm reduction, and reinsertion inhibit a different implementation problem. The legislation regarding these activities does not oblige communities to implement the law. The law rather sets a framework for those communities that wish to undertake such activities—it is an enabling law. For example, the law sets rules for shooting rooms: their size and the facilities and personnel needed. Therefore, the law will enable those who were already thinking about harm reduction activities to take the opportunity to bring their ideas into practice, but those who have not thought about harm reduction yet either say it is not their responsibility or are at a loss because they have no clue how to bring the law into practice.

In conclusion, Portugal has deliberately set forth on a novel approach to dealing with the problems of drug use that is consistent with a set of general humanistic and pragmatic principles and consistent with international laws and treaties. This approach will be followed carefully and, if successful, could lead to significant changes in the way many nations approach drug policy.

References

Assembleia da República. 2000. *Define o regime jurídico applicável ao consumo de estupefaciantes e substáncias psicotrópicas, bem como a protecção sanitária e social das pessoas que consomem tais substáncias sem prescrição médica*. Lei no. 30/2000. Lisboa, Portugal: Assembleia da República, Depósito Legal.

Banco de Portugal. 2001. *Relatório Anual de 2000*. Lisboa, Portugal: Banco de Portugal.

Comissão para a Estratégia Nacional de Combate à Droga. 1998. *Estratégia nacional de luta contra a droga*. Lisboa, Portugal. Mimeographed.

Conselho de Ministros. 2000. *Plano de acção nacional de luta contra a droga e a toxicodependência—Horizonte 2004.* Lisboa: Government of Portugal.

European Monitoring Center on Drugs and Drug Addiction (EMCDDA). 2001. *Complementary statistical tables to the 2000 annual report on the state of the drugs problem in the European Union.* Lisboa, Portugal: European Monitoring Center on Drugs and Drug Addiction.

Government of Portugal. 1999. *Resolution of the Council of Ministers no. 46/ 99.* 22 April. Lisboa: Government of Portugal, Depósito Legal.

———. 2000. *National drug strategy* (officially translated from Portuguese to English). Depósito legal no. 148314/ 00. Lisboa: Government of Portugal, Depósito Legal.

Instituto Português da Droga e da Toxicodependência (IPDT). 2000. *National strategies: Institutional and legal frameworks.* Lisboa, Portugal: Instituto Português da Droga e da Toxicodependência.

Kahan, J. P., M. van het Loo, M. Franco, J. G. Cravinho, V. Rato, J. T. Silveira, and F. Fonseca. 1999. *A seminar game to analyze regional governance options for Portugal.* Report no. MR-1031-RE/ FLAD. Santa Monica, CA: RAND.

Sechrest, D. K., and D. Shicor, eds. 2001. Drug courts as an alternative treatment modality. Special issue. *Journal of Drug Issues* 31 (1).

Serviço de Prevenção e Tratamento da Toxicodependência (SPTT). 1999. *Relatório de actividades 1999, Versão abreviada.* Lisboa, Portugal: Serviço de Prevenção e Tratamento da Toxicodependência.

van het Loo, M., J. P. Kahan, J.A.K. Cave, and C. Meijer. 2000. *Measuring the roles, structures and cooperation of drug demand reduction services: Results of a preliminary study.* EMCDDA report no. CT.99.TR.01. Lisboa, Portugal: European Monitoring Center on Drugs and Drug Addiction.

ANNALS, *AAPSS*, **582**, July 2002

Swedish Drug Policy in the Twenty-First Century: A Policy Model Going Astray

By LEIF LENKE and BOERJE OLSSON

ABSTRACT: During the 1990s, the drug problem in Sweden stabilized in spite of a heroin wave on the European continent and in the United Kingdom. The preconditions for this control policy are discussed, as are the advantages of the Swedish drug control model with its massiveness regarding prevention, treatment, and repression. When drawing conclusions from the 1980's, focus has been placed on zero tolerance and dissociation of harm reduction activities in connection with the economic crisis that, although temporary, hit Swedish society in the 1990s. This resulted in the control policy's having a list so that preventive measures and treatment had to give in on behalf of further strengthening of the police in the drug control model. The change in focus toward an even more pronounced zero tolerance approach did not yield any visible results regarding drug use. Experimenting with drugs and heavy drug use increased considerably during the 1990s.

Leif Lenke is a full professor of criminology.

Boerje Olsson is a full professor of social alcohol and drug research. Both are active at Stockholm University, have taken part in the buildup of European drug policy and drug epidemiology networks, and have presented comparative analyses of European drug problems.

NOTE: We would like to thank Mikael Nilsson at the Ministry of Justice for his valuable contributions to the analyses in this article.

A T the peak of the Swedish euphoria regarding its claimed successful drug policy in the beginning of the 1990s, a report from a governmental task force was given the title "We Never Give Up!" (1991). The tone of the report is optimistic but includes a few sentences that illustrate the swing that had taken place in the earlier welfare-society-based Swedish drug policy. The police representative formulated a thought that would probably not have been accepted in such a report ten years earlier. He wrote,

We disturb them [the drug users] in their activities, and threaten them with compulsory treatment and make their life difficult. It *shall* be difficult to be a drug misuser. The more difficult we make their living, the more clear the other alternative, i.e., a drug free life, will appear. (P. 14)

This formulation illustrates how the focus had been systematically shifted from a perspective of drug misuse as a social problem with social roots to a substance-fixated approach where the police organization naturally was—and should be— given the central role in the new drug policy. This approach spilled over to the social welfare authorities as well, and to demand a drug-free lifestyle before providing treatment and other social welfare services is a common practice in Sweden today.

Unfortunately, in the 1990s, this was shown to be a serious mistake (Olsson et al. 2001; SOU 2000, 126) that still casts its shadow over the Swedish drug policy of the beginning the new millennium.

This article provides an overview of Swedish drug policy and places it in a political and social context. A further objective is to make use of a comparative perspective to make the reading easier to grasp for non-Swedish and particularly non-European readers. The article employs a historical approach, and aspects of both the drug problem and drug policy are described in chronological order.

THE 1960s— A PERIOD OF OPTIONS

During the 1960s, Sweden benefited from having been able to avoid becoming entangled in the war. The economy was booming due to the great demand for Swedish industrial products needed to rebuild Europe. Politically, Sweden was a stable society with a low degree of political polarization. The Social Democrats had been the dominant political party since the 1930s, and parties on the radical Left as well as on the radical Right were marginalized. The largest opposition party was the Liberal Party and not the Conservatives, but this latter group, as will be described below, successively strengthened its position and took the lead by the end of the century. Civil society was strong and was supported by a tight structure of organizations such as labor unions, farmers' organizations, and people's movements such as the temperance movement, tenant organizations, and so forth.

*The drug question
during the 1960s*

To the surprise of many, the affluent welfare society did not eradicate crime and social problems as many had believed quite strongly that it would prior to World War II. Instead, crime rates soared during the postwar period and a number of youth cultures developed.

The challenges that drug use and drug problems pose to a particular society are dependent not only on specific developments in drug patterns and trends but also on any peculiarities in a society's historical, moral, and social contexts. To understand Swedish drug problems and policies, at least some of these factors must be highlighted. One such factor that is often striking to non-Swedish observers is the long historical dominance of amphetamines, as opposed to heroin, as the substance of choice among problem drug users.

The legal use of amphetamines did not constitute, or at least was not defined as, a social problem during the decades preceding the 1960s. Beneath the surface, however, a process had started that would transform or redefine drug use from being an individual medical problem to being a public social/legal problem. The widespread availability of amphetamines constituted one necessary precondition, while the incorporation of this substance into the criminal subculture constituted another and definitively triggered the public concern (Olsson 1994).

Until the first half of the 1960s, the medical profession actively fought to maintain traditional medical definitions of drug problems.

They struggled to combat initiatives whose aim was to introduce stiffer sanctions against drug-related activities. As it was framed at the time, such a course of action was felt to be tantamount to criminalizing an illness. Traditional medical remedies were, however, not capable of curing what were obviously social problems, and by the mid-1960s, the medical community had withdrawn from the public discourse around the drug issue (Olsson 1994).

The subcultural use of amphetamines, however, continued to grow, and as more coherent drug policy measures were put together, international youth trends meant that cannabis was also becoming popular among Swedish youth, which transformed what had been a general anxiety into something approaching a public panic. Experimental drug use among the young peaked in the early 1970s and subsequently followed a decreasing trend that lasted until the final years of the 1980s. The remaining years of the twentieth century were characterized by an increasing trend that had yet (in 1999) to reach a peak (see Figure 1).

In the 1960s, Sweden actually went as far as trying a prescription program that probably went even further than the programs developed in the United Kingdom under the so-called British model of the 1960s. One hundred forty clients were prescribed large doses of amphetamines as well as opiates. The program was halted after eighteen months with regard to the very liberal prescription practice.[1] The project was "evaluated"[2] by Nils Bejerot, who would later play an important role in the

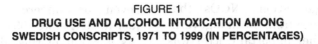

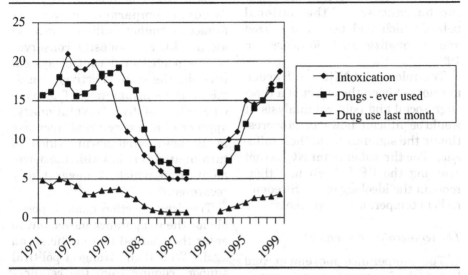

Swedish drug policy debate. The project was labeled a catastrophe and the cause of the Swedish drug epidemic.

In spite of the indisputably very liberal prescription practice, the Swedish Drug Treatment Commission of 1969 came to the conclusion that the program had not reduced criminality (other than drug crimes) in a significant way. On the other hand, it did not claim that the program had had negative consequences as regards the recruitment of new drug users, a conclusion that was confirmed later in a reevaluation of the program (Lenke and Olsson 1998a).

THE 1970s—
RECONSTRUCTION "FROM BELOW"

The 1970s in Sweden were a period of transition. The very strong economic growth that had placed Sweden among the top nations in relation to per capita GNP came up against external problems. The oil crisis and the structural problems experienced by the shipping industry, for example, led to the first—albeit limited—youth unemployment since World War II.

In the political arena, the Social Democrats lost ground. An agrarian party (the Center Party) gained more than 20 percent of the votes, and for the first time since the 1930s, a coalition of the Center-Right was voted into office in 1976, which then governed until 1982.

During the 1970s, the drug question successively assumed an increasingly central position in the political arena. The drug issue was successfully socially constructed. Central actors in this process were a number of grassroots nongovernmental organizations (NGOs) that gained support from the new government. Another important actor was the bureaucracy of the national police, which had been centralized and nationalized in 1965 (Kassman 1998).[3]

The role of the NGOs in Sweden has not yet been the object of a thorough social and political analysis. It would be difficult, however, to overestimate the significance of their influence. The three dominant NGOs (not counting the RFHL[4]) all had their roots in the ideology of the Sweden's radical temperance movements.

The temperance movement

The temperance movement had lost much of its once very strong position in Swedish society through its support of the abolition of the alcohol rationing system in 1955. This may seem a little odd to non-Swedish readers, but it is related to the movement's strict zero tolerance or prohibitionist profile. That the state produced and distributed alcohol and thus legitimized the alcohol culture was not acceptable to the radical branches of the temperance movement. This stands in sharp contrast to the more moderate temperance movements on the European continent (including Denmark), which chose to view the alcohol question from a public health perspective—rather than as a moral issue—and focused on liquor as the major alcohol problem. The Swedish radical temperance movement instead—like their allies in Finland, Norway, and Iceland as well as in North America—saw beer as the stepping-stone to hard liquor and thus sometimes as

an even more dangerous enemy than liquor itself (Lenke 1991).

As a result of this ideology, the Swedish temperance movement formed an "unholy" alliance with the alcohol liberals—mostly conservatives—to abolish a control system whereby the state effectively legitimized the consumption of alcohol. One effect of this "revolutionary" approach was a very sizable increase in alcohol-related harm, which in turn created a crisis within the movement from which it never really recovered.

The drug question made it possible for the temperance movement to enter the political and public arena again. With their strongest political support coming from the center—particularly the Liberals—they were now able to make progress once again. As a consequence, Sweden witnessed the introduction of the first new alcohol restrictions for many decades, including among other things a prohibition on the sale of strong beer in grocery stores. As is discussed below, the revival of the temperance movement—even if only temporary—may also have been a significant event in relation to the drug question.

The drug control NGOs

The various drug control NGOs had different profiles. One was an organization for the parents of drug users that fought, among other things, for compulsory treatment programs for drug users. Such a course of action had hitherto been an option only for the treatment of alcohol abusers.

Another movement is the Hassela Solidarity Organization, with political ties to the Social Democrats. The National Association for a Drug Free Society has also been an important player. This movement, and to some extent the others as well, have as their ideological father a medical doctor, Nils Bejerot, whose ideological roots lay in the authoritarian Left and the Swedish temperance movement. He worked for the Swedish police as a medical expert and played a central role in the strategy to involve the police in the "crusade" to convince both the public and politicians that the drug question should be resolved in a certain way. As models of a successful strategy, he looked to the situation in Japan in the 1950s as well as to China's drug policy during the postrevolutionary period (i.e., transportation to labor camps).

By the end of the 1970s, it is reasonable to say that Swedish drug policy had shifted its profile. The focus had moved from international syndicates and the treatment of "drug victims" to a police-oriented strategy whose objective was to clear the streets of drug pushers. These were to be placed in compulsory treatment to stop this "contagious disease," which is how drug use was portrayed to the public. From then on, all forms of possession of drugs were to be prosecuted and were to lead to at least a fine.

Compulsory treatment for adult drug users—which was one of the central demands made by the NGOs—was introduced in the early 1980s. The time limits, however, were rather restricted (maximum six months), and the main purpose of this type of treatment was to motivate drug users to undergo treatment in other forms.

The high profile of the drug question was thus cemented, and massive preventive programs were launched by means of which people were made to believe that drug use was the root of many social problems like criminal careers, prostitution, HIV, and so forth.[5] In an opinion poll of 1980, 46 percent reported drug misuse to be the social problem that worried them most (Olsson 1994, 1). In another poll of 1984, 95 percent thought drug use should be criminalized.

The same government also revived the activities of the—at that time rather passive—European drug control collaboration conducted within the framework of the so-called Pompidou Group.[6] This was achieved by joining with Norway in the provision of economic resources (and by moving the group from the European Community to the Council of Europe, where Sweden and Norway were members).

In "the problem stream," to quote Kingdon (1984), heroin was introduced on the Swedish market, and amphetamine use had been spread outside the big cities. The peak in drug use in general, however, took place already in the beginning of the 1970s.

THE 1980s—
TOWARD ZERO TOLERANCE

The 1980s in Sweden have been characterized as the decade of the right-wing wave in politics. In the case of Sweden, however, this did not mean that everybody started to vote for right-wing parties. It should rather be seen as a slow process whereby all the political parties took steps toward more right-wing positions. This swing in politics was undoubtedly influenced by the conservative successes of President Reagan in the United States and Prime Minister Thatcher in the United Kingdom.

The Social Democrats regained power in the 1982 elections, however, and fulfilled their promise to set up a governmental commission on the drug question. During the election campaign, the Social Democrats had already taken a tough stance to regain the initiative in the drug question. There was no new drug policy, however. A new and more pragmatic political process had started that might reasonably be referred to as "tango politics." This term describes a political process wherein one party—in this case the Social Democrats—first "lost" the political discourse on how to handle the drug question. When the treatment-first approach was defeated by the Conservatives' repression-first approach, the Social Democrats successively positioned themselves as close to the Conservative perspective as possible, hoping that the voters would no longer be able to see which party was really "leading the dance."

The commission's rhetoric was tough, but they in fact made only limited concessions to the repressive position. Penal law was strengthened marginally, but the commission did not recommend the criminalization of the mere use of drugs, as the opposition parties demanded.

After intense attacks from both the political opposition and the NGOs, including organized marches from the countryside to Stockholm with antidrug banners flying, the Social Democratic minister of justice gave in and criminalized drug use in 1988. The sanction was limited to a small fine.

The opposition campaign continued, arguing that mere criminalization was not enough. The imposition of a prison sanction was called for, as this would make it possible to impose urine tests. In a bill presented to the Swedish parliament of 1989-1990 (m 511), the Conservatives once again demanded heavier penalties, including life imprisonment for aggravated drug offences.

In the middle of the 1980s, the AIDS question surfaced in Sweden, taking an extremely alarmist form.[7] A panic-like situation developed, as the new disease threatened to spread from the sexually very active intravenous amphetamine population to the general public. Extraordinary restrictive measures were imposed to control the spread of the disease.[8] At the same time, however, a massive program was put in place to identify all drug users, to motivate them to get tested, and to offer them drug treatment (primarily on a voluntary basis).

This offensive drug policy came to be seen as the Swedish drug control model and gained wide recognition as it had a profile that corresponded well with the Swedish welfare perspective. It combined the extensive use of treatment with massive control measures in a social and political environment where marginalization and poverty were at their lowest levels ever. At the same time, full employment, housing, and decent programs for refugees were at hand as never before and with few competitors abroad. Thus, the drug policy was implemented in an extraordinarily positive social period.

THE 1990s—
RECONSTRUCTION "FROM ABOVE"

The context changed quite dramatically at the beginning of the 1990s. Sweden, which had managed to avoid the policies of the European Union with its more than 20 percent youth unemployment rates, went into a deep economic crisis. The second non–Social Democratic government since World War II was voted into power in 1992, and unemployment rose rapidly.[9] The economic crisis created an enormous budget deficit that had repercussions for almost all public activities, with the public sector taking the brunt of the inevitable cutbacks. Treatment facilities, schools, hospitals, and community programs directed at the support of young people were cut drastically, and youth unemployment rose from 2 percent to almost 15 percent during a period of four years.

The new government also fulfilled its election promise to impose a prison sentence (maximum six months) for the use of drugs. This new level of sanction allowed the police to use extraordinary measures to secure evidence. In this case, it meant they were able to impose compulsory urine and blood tests on suspected drug users.[10]

The Swedish war on drugs now reached its peak, and the rhetoric started to level off.[11] The new Swedish government institutionalized its own policy by creating a new control bureaucracy to take the lead in the implementation of drug policy in Sweden—the National Board of Public Health.[12] This organization immediately profiled itself by organizing a conference and inviting an American Drug Enforcement Administration agent to outline drug policy priorities. It was no surprise that this speech was devoid of anything that might suggest to the listener that drug policy had anything whatsoever to do with social welfare. The focus was exclusively on control measures and the dissemination of information.

The new organization also produced a white book in four languages to describe the "successful Swedish control model" and to present the model to an international, and particularly a European, audience.

It is interesting to notice that this first white book on Swedish drug policy in 1993 did not mention social welfare as a relevant factor in Swedish drug policy (Swedish National Board for Public Health [SNBPH] 1993). In the 1998 version (under the Social Democratic government), however, social welfare is strongly emphasized. It says in a special section called "Drug Policy/Part and Parcel of Welfare Policy" that "a restrictive drug policy must go hand in hand with a policy that does not allow unemployment, segregation and social distress to grow" (SNBPH 1998, 8).

A kind of natural experiment had suddenly been created. The repressive aspects of drug control policy were maximized at the same time as the role played by other aspects of drug policy (which had often been ridiculed as "flower-powerish" in the context of the political discourse) was reduced.

The experiment was not a success. All indicators relating to all categories of drug use began to climb along a curve that has not yet reached a peak.

ANALYSES

The low level of drug use in general

The level of drug use in Sweden is without doubt relatively low from an international perspective. The prevalence of having used cannabis during the past year in Sweden is 1 percent of the general population. For countries with more liberal drug policies, figures are higher: Denmark at 4 percent and the Netherlands at 5 percent. Some countries are on even higher levels, with Spain at 7 percent and the United Kingdom at 9 percent (European Monitoring Center on Drugs and Drug Addiction 2000).

A closer look at specific categories of drug use indicates that the picture is not quite so clear-cut, however. As regards heavy drug use, indicated by the regular use of any drug or any use of intravenous drugs, the picture is not so clear. Case-finding studies are notoriously problematic when it comes to cross-national comparisons, and indicators of heavy drug use—such as drug-related deaths, for example—give a rather unclear picture.

Perhaps one conclusion can be established. The use of heroin—particularly intravenous heroin use—is comparatively rare in Sweden. It is not easy to explain the Swedish preference for intravenous amphetamine use, which has no correspondence in Europe. It appears, however, that the early establishment of a culture of intravenous amphetamine use may have had some kind of protective effect with regard to the use of heroin. There are clear indications that (intravenous) amphetamine users have regarded heroin use as something strange and dangerous. Studies of drug-related deaths confirm this picture to some extent since death rates are much lower for this category of drug use.

It is quite possibly also the case that the rather widespread use of amphetamines functions in competition with the much more expensive use of cocaine, with the result that up to now, the market for cocaine has been very limited in Sweden.

Drug-using cultures in Sweden have also shown a strong tendency to concentrate into isolated subcultures so that in spite of the existence of heroin cultures in both Stockholm and Malmo (close to Copenhagen), it took twenty-five years before a heroin epidemic hit Gothenburg,[13] which is a city double the size of Malmo and situated between the other two cities.

Another protective factor in the Swedish case is the country's geopolitical position. A study of heroin seizures in Europe has shown that a peripheral position (i.e., Eire, Norway, Sweden, Finland) in relation to the broad streams of heroin traffic in Europe (from the Balkans to Northern Europe) functioned as a protection against heroin misuse. Swedish social policy, particularly policies focused on combating youth unemployment, has served as an additional protective factor (Lenke and Olsson 1996 and 1998b).

One characteristic specific to the Swedish drug problem has been the extensive overlap with other social problems. There appears to be a very considerable overlap, for example, between the amphetamine epidemic and the population of "early onset juvenile delinquents" (von Hofer, Lenke, and Thorsson 1983; Olsson 1994). Thus, the introduction of intravenous amphetamine use in Sweden did not increase the risk of engaging in a criminal career across different birth cohorts. This led to the conclusion that narcotic drugs rather transformed the careers from early onset of general social problems, delinquency, and heavy alcohol use to an even more problematic career, and narcotic drugs were added to the criminal career profile, this without extending the size of the marginalized group.

Extensive overlaps of this kind are not reported from nations on the European continent, where heavy drug use is found to a significant extent in other social strata as well.

Finally, one group at risk of becoming heavy drug users in many European countries has been immigrants, especially second-generation immigrants. This group has been rather well integrated into Swedish society, however, and presents lower crime rates than first-generation immigrants, for example.[14] This constitutes a positive idiosyncrasy in comparison to most other countries in Europe. Up until the 1990s, immigrants had not been overrepresented in the population of heavy drug users.

The temperance question

Another factor that must be assigned a central role in relation to patterns of drug use in Sweden is the remains of the influence from a long and strong tradition of temperance. Traces of this tradition are still to be found in Swedish alcohol policy, and when it comes to the rather strong short-term decrease in juvenile drug use in the 1980s, the explanation is most probably to be found in the alcohol political activities launched at the end of the 1970s.

Longitudinal surveys of drinking and drug habits among military conscripts have shown that drinking to intoxication has been a strong predictive factor for later experimentation with narcotic drugs. Around 15 percent of conscripts report regularly drinking to the point of intoxication (see Figure 1). Around 50 percent of those who have ever tried drugs are recruited from this group. For the more regular drug users, the figure is around 60 percent.

As can be seen from Figure 1, the rapid decrease in drug use during the 1980s was preceded by a corresponding decrease in drinking to the point of intoxication. Other empirical findings also suggest that it was the extensive integrated antialcohol and antidrug program rather than the police crackdown that resulted in the drop in drug use. Thus, it was not just alcohol and drug use, but glue sniffing, that followed the U-shaped curve in the 1980s. Nobody has ever claimed that the police crackdown might have anything to do with the patterns of drinking to the point of intoxication[15] (Lenke and Olsson 2000).

As can also be seen from Figure 1, all these begin to climb again at the beginning of the 1990s. The reason for this will be discussed below in relation to developments in the party political arena.

A "symbolic crusade"?

To understand the heat of the Swedish drug policy debate, it would be helpful to draw one or two parallels to Gusfield's (1980) study of the American prohibition movements of the early twentieth century. There are many indications, for example, that Swedish drug policy was not a policy created from above—as it was in the United States during the Nixon administration (Sharp 1994, 16).[16]

It is more reasonable to interpret developments here as a process whereby the rural community in Sweden was making a final effort to regain control over the process of modernization, globalization, Europeanization, and the centralization of capital. The NGOs described above all had a stronger basis of support outside the big cities, and their programs stated quite explicitly that modern youth lifestyles (including drug use) were the main targets of their activities.[17]

The partisan dimension of drug policy

The NGOs, however, would not have succeeded so easily without the support of party political processes that had been stirred into action by their activities. When the Conservatives added drug policy to their law-and-order agenda, however, a peculiar process was set in motion. In sharp contrast to the more drug-liberal countries on the European continent, where the Conservatives who had been in power when drug policy was formulated chose to treat drug problems in the same way as alcohol problems, that is, as individual problems with the medical profession's providing the "solution," the Swedish Conservatives handed the drug issue over to the police, an organization well prepared to compete for more resources and social prestige.

When the Social Democrats responded with the strategy of tango politics as described above, the spiral did not turn into an open confrontation as quickly as it might have. The price that Sweden paid, however, was that the public debate focused on the drug problem withered away. As this strategy gave the impression of an absolute national consensus,[18] the media also dropped their critical stance in relation to the drug issue and started instead to function as a public address system for official policy and the police. A climate was created in the public debate that led one author to describe the Swedish drug policy as having gradually developed into a "national project," functioning to strengthen falling levels of social cohesion in a time of globalization (Tham 1995).

Researchers and other drug policy experts were in many ways placed in intellectual quarantine where they remain to this day. If experts bring up the drug question, the NGOs are inevitably awakened and take the opportunity to exploit space in the media to demand new restrictions from the politicians. The political parties either try to avoid the topic—the left-wing parties—or take the opportunity to gain votes—the Conservatives—by sharpening their law-and-order profile. Thus, the incentives for experts to try to introduce relevant facts into the debate are rather limited. One consequence is that public awareness slowly withers away, and anything can be presented as a fact in the debate without the risk of scrutiny.

Ignorance on the part of the media is the rule when it comes to attempts to inject a more nuanced picture of the problem into the drug control discourse. In the television media, the setting is even more problematic. To make a drug policy debate interesting, experts are invited exclusively in the role of full-blown legalizers and are forced to do combat with an NGO gladiator without the slightest requirement to keep to any rules of objectiveness and so forth.

There are many indications that the integration of the drug question into the law-and-order policy arena was a very fruitful strategy for the Conservatives. Until the 1970s, the non-Socialist wing of Swedish politics had been dominated by the Center and Liberal parties. By contrast with the Conservatives, these parties supported the temperance movement. In the course of the so-called

right-wing wave of the 1980s, however, the Conservatives outmaneuvered their fellow bourgeois parties. The Conservatives' very strong focus on the issue of law and order was most probably an important factor in this process.

Because of the strong focus on narcotic drugs—and thus no longer on the alcohol and drug question as a single integrated issue as it had been viewed during the 1970s—the Conservatives gained momentum. Since the Conservatives faced no real competition on the law-and-order question, the Center-Liberals invited the Conservatives to take the hegemonic position over the political right wing. As a consequence, the Center-Liberals lost the political strength to support not only the withering temperance movements but also the other social groups who were fighting the symbolic crusade described above.

FINAL REMARKS

There is an obvious risk of falling into a state of cynicism when discussing problems such as those described above. It should, however, be noted that there are some areas of light in the otherwise rather grim picture. There are a number of facts that should be added to this picture. Swedish drug policy is not the most repressive in Europe, for example. Maximum prison terms are higher in almost every other European country. The maximum penalty for drug crimes is imprisonment for ten years compared, for example, to fifteen years in Germany, sixteen years in the Netherlands, twenty years in

Spain, and thirty years in France and Italy (Dorn and Jamieson 2000, 9), and the Swedish prison population has not increased as a consequence of drug policy. This is in stark contrast to the situation in the Netherlands, for example, where the prison population has almost tripled during the past fifteen years.[19]

Another point is that the NGOs have never demanded draconian punishments and have not always supported demands from the police organization to be given extraordinary powers. Thus, the use of hidden microphones (bugging) is not permitted, nor are the police allowed to provoke people into committing drug offences. There is still no registration—outside of police arrest and conviction records—of drug users in Sweden, as can be found in the United Kingdom, for example. Nor are there any extreme rules of forfeiture.

It is unclear which direction drug policy will take in the future. A report published recently by a government commission, the Drugs Commission, titled *The Choice—The Drug Policy Challenge* provides an example of the confrontation between reality and idealistic visions. The commission stated that "there are big deficiencies in the area of drug policy" (Narkotikakommissionen 2000, 11). These deficiencies, however, are not related to the way in which the basic principles behind Swedish drug policies have been formulated during the past twenty years. The problems are seen almost entirely as consequences of cutbacks in public sector funding. The main conclusion drawn by the commission is that "Sweden's restrictive policy must be sustained and reinforced" (Narkotikakommissionen 2000, 11). It is also important to emphasize the fact that according to its terms of reference, the commission was to stick with the basic principles of a restrictive drug policy and the goal of a drug-free society. In this respect, no reconsideration was allowed. In summary, drug policy as it has already been formulated is still perceived as the best possible. It is simply a matter of restoring it to its former glory. The question, however, is whether the reality that drug policy has to cope with is the same today as it was ten years ago.

One thing seems to be clear, however. A policy that once had been formulated from below has been taken over by the political establishment and is today to a very large extent steered from above. In this sense, the direction of Swedish drug policy has more in common with that of the United States than merely the zero tolerance approach.

Notes

1. The clients had a strong say in the size of their doses as the program was given under a nonauthoritarian model.

2. This evaluation was later checked with the use of modern time-series, which did not corroborate Bejerot's results.

3. Eisner (1997), after having read our analysis of the strength and central role in the Swedish drug policy discourse, came to the conclusion that Switzerland would never have had its heroin prescription program materialized if its police forces had been centralized.

4. RFHL is a client organization for drug users established in 1965.

5. The parallels with the heyday of the temperance movement at the beginning of the twentieth century, when alcohol was said to be the root of almost all social problems, includ-

ing poverty, sickness, crime, illegitimate births, and so forth, are striking.

6. The Council of Europe is an organization of European nations. The Pompidou Group is a group of political representatives from each nation who meet annually to discuss and coordinate European drug policy. The Pompidou Group was established in the early 1970s by French President Pompidou as a gesture to meet the wishes of President Nixon after the revelation of the French connection in drug trafficking to the United States.

7. The most alarmist book was published by an institute directed by Nils Bejerot, mentioned above.

8. Sweden, in a comparative study of European countries, stands out as the country with the strongest emphasis on control of HIV programs and also individual HIV patients (Panchaud 1995, 81).

9. It is fair to say that the new government has not been blamed for the economic crisis, not even by the Social Democrats. Perhaps it has been blamed more for letting the recession go so deep.

10. Such tests have since been used at the rate of about ten thousand per year, which is also the number of persons arrested for crimes according to the drug legislation.

11. The Conservative party has, however, asked for life imprisonment as a maximum punishment for drug crimes.

12. Bertram et al. (1996, 107, 126) reported a similar party political institutionalization of the American drug policy with the creation of the Drug Enforcement Administration by President Nixon in 1973.

13. The reason for the epidemic's reaching Gothenburg is probably to be found in the fact that a new "pipe-line," to quote Reuter and Kleiman (1986), had been installed to supply the Norwegian heroin market. The heavy drug use problem in Norway has been dominated by heroin instead of the amphetamines that dominate in Sweden.

14. In 1999, 1 million of Sweden's 9 million inhabitants were born abroad. A third were born in Scandinavia (mainly Finland), and a third in the rest of Europe. In the 1980s and 1990s, around 250,000 immigrants arrived from Asia (mainly Iran, Iraq, and Turkey), and 50,000 from South America and Africa each.

15. Glue sniffing shows the same development.

16. Sharp (1994) used the term "mobilization model."

17. This interpretation differs partly from that of Boekhout van Solinge's (1997), for example, who sees drug control policy in Sweden as a sign of "general backwardness" in the periphery of Europe. In fact, Sweden had an "endemic" intravenous epidemic many years before the Netherlands did.

18. This should not hide the fact that there is a strong consensus in Swedish drug policy. As mentioned above, there are, however, significant nuances when it comes to the relevance of social welfare factors as a precondition for the construction of drug policy.

19. The Dutch prison population rose from 20 to 84 per 100,000 inhabitants between 1975 and 1999, compared to a rise from 55 to 60 in Sweden (Home Office Statistical Bulletin 2000). An important reason for the Dutch increase is the increase in drug-related crimes and stiffer punishments for drug crimes in the Netherlands (von Hofer 1998, 166, referring to Dutch sources). (Corresponding rates for the United States are above 700.)

References

Bertram, E., M. Blachman, K. Sharpe, and P. Andreas. 1996. *Drug war politics: The price of denial*. Berkeley: University of California Press.

Boekhout van Solinge, T. 1997. *The Swedish drug control system: An in-depth review and analysis*. Amsterdam: Jan Mets. Cedro.

Dorn, N., and A. Jamieson. 2000. *European drug laws: The room for manoeuvre*. London: DrugScope.

Eisner, M. 1997. Determinants of Swiss drug policy: The case of the heroin prescription program. *Journal of Drug Issues* (July).

European Monitoring Center on Drugs and Drug Addiction. 2000. *Annual report on the state of the drug problem in the European Union*. Lisboa, Portugal: European Monitoring Center on Drugs and Drug Addiction.

Gusfield, J. R. 1980. *Symbolic crusade: Status politics and the American tem-*

perance movement. Westport, CT: Greenwood.

Home Office Statistical Bulletin 2000. London.

Kassman, A. 1997. *Polisen och narkotikaproblemet: från nationella aktioner mot narkotikaprofitörer till lokala insatser för att stoera missbruket* (The police and the drug problem). Stockholm: Almqvist & Wiksell International.

Kingdon, J. W. 1984. *Agendas, alternatives, and public policies*. London: Scott, Foresman.

Lenke. L. 1991. Dryckesmoenster, nykterhetsroerelser och narkotikapolitik—en analys av samspelet mellan bruk av droger, brukets konsekvenser och formerna foer deras kontroll i ett historiskt och komparativt perspektiv (The significance of distilled beverages—Reflections on the formation of drinking cultures and anti-drug movements). *Sociologisk forskning*. Nr 4/91.

Lenke, L., and B. Olsson. 1996. Sweden: Zero tolerance wins the argument? In *European drug policies and enforcement*, edited by N. Dorn, J. Jepsen, and E. Savona. London: Wiltshire, Macmillan.

———. 1998a. Drugs on prescription—The Swedish experiment of 1965-67 in retrospect. *European Addiction Research* 4: 183-89.

———. 1998b. Heroin seizures as an indicator of variation in market situations, drug availability and heroin use in Europe. Report to the Pompidou Group, Council of Europe, Strasbourg, France. Mimeographed.

———. 2000. Swedish drug policy in perspective. In *Current and future drug policies in Europe: Problems, prospects and research methods*, edited by H.-J. Albrecht, A. Kalmthout, and J. Derks. Freiburg, Germany: Max Planck Institute for International and Comparative Criminal Law.

Narkotikakommissionen 2000. Drug Policy Commission. SOU 2000:126. *Vaegvalet - Den narkotikapolitiska utmaningen*.

Narkotikakommissionen 2000. Drug Policy Commission. SOU 2000:126. *Vaegvalet - Den narkotikapolitiska utmaningen*.

Olsson, B. 1994. Narkotikaproblemets bakgrund (The background of the drug problem.) Ph.D. diss., The Swedish Council for Information on Alcohol and Other Drugs, CAN. Stockholm.

Olsson, B., C. Adamsson-Wahren, and S. Byqvist. 2001. Det tunga narkotikamissbrukets omfattning i Sverige 1998 (Heavy drug use in Sweden 1998). The Swedish Council for Information on Alcohol and Other Drugs, CAN. Stockholm.

Panchaud, C. 1995. Welfare states facing HIV/AIDS: Organizational responses in Western Europe (1981-91). *Swiss Political Science Review* 1 (4): 65-94.

Reuter, P., and M. Kleiman. 1986. Risk and prices: An economic analysis of drug enforcement. In *Crime and justice*, vol. 7, edited by M. Tonry and N. Morris, 289-339. Chicago: University of Chicago Press.

Sharp, E. 1994. *The dilemma of drug policy in the United States*. New York: HarperCollins.

Swedish National Board for Public Health (SNBPH). 1993. *The Swedish experience*. Stockholm: Swedish National Board for Public Health.

———. 1998. *A preventive strategy*. Stockholm: Swedish National Board for Public Health.

Tham, H. 1995. Drug control as a national project: The case of Sweden. *Journal of Drug Issues* 25 (1): 113-28.

von Hofer, H., L. Lenke, and U. Thorsson. 1983. Criminality among 13 Swedish

Birth Cohorts. *Brit. J. Criminology* 23(3):263-69.

von Hofer, H. 1998. Fangtal och kriminalpolitik i Holland och Sverige (Prison rates and crime policy in Holland and Sweden). In *Brottsligheten i Europa* (Crime in Europe), edited by H. von Hofer. Lund. Studentlitteratur.

"We never give up! " (Vi ger oss aldrig!). 1991 Report from a governmental task force. Stockholm.

ANNALS, *AAPSS*, **582**, July 2002

Harm Minimization in a Prohibition Context—Australia

By GABRIELE BAMMER, WAYNE HALL, MARGARET HAMILTON, and ROBERT ALI

ABSTRACT: Australia ranks high internationally in the prevalence of cannabis and other illicit drug use, with the prevalence of all illicit drug use increasing since the 1970s. There are two distinctive features associated with harms from injecting drug use—high rates of death from heroin overdose and low rates of HIV infection. Australia has largely avoided a punitive and moralistic drug policy, developing instead harm minimization strategies and a robust treatment framework embedded in a strong law enforcement regime. Two illustrations of Australian drug policy are presented: legislation that provides for the expiation of simple cannabis offences by payment of a fine and the widespread implementation of agonist maintenance treatment for heroin dependence.

Gabriele Bammer is a senior fellow at the National Centre for Epidemiology and Population Health at the Australian National University. She directed feasibility research into an Australian heroin trial and has subsequently been involved in trialing other treatments for heroin dependence.

Wayne Hall is now professor and director of the Office of Public Policy and Ethics at the Insitute of Molecular Bioscence. Until September 2001, he was director of the National Drug and Alcohol Research Centre, University of New South Wales.

Margaret Hamilton is director of Turning Point, an alcohol and drug research, policy and program development centre affiliated with The University of Melbourne. She has more than thirty years experience in this field including treatment and prevention evaluation research, and serves on many national and state policy advisory bodies.

Robert Ali is a public health physician who is currently the director of Clinical Policy & Research at the Drug & Alcohol Services Council of South Australia. He is also member of the Cochrane Alcohol and Drug groups editorial board.

AN OVERVIEW OF
AUSTRALIA'S DRUG PROBLEMS

General background

Australia is a sparsely populated island continent of increasingly heterogeneous national origins. Cannabis is grown around Australia, both as hydroponic indoor crops and in a range of secluded locations. There is legal poppy cultivation for the pharmaceutical industry in the southernmost island state of Tasmania but no evidence of diversion or of illegal cultivation. There is no evidence of cocaine cultivation. There is production throughout Australia of amphetamine derivatives and analogues with the exception of 3,4methylene-dioxymethylamphetamine (MDMA, or ecstasy), which is more complicated to manufacture. There is also significant importation of cannabis, heroin, cocaine, amphetamines, and MDMA. Despite 25,760 kilometers of coastline, both intelligence and seizures suggest that most drugs are imported through Sydney, a busy international and domestic port for people, mail, and cargo. As Australia's largest city, with a population of around 4 million people, it also offers a degree of anonymity.

Most drug users accessing treatment come from Anglo-Australian backgrounds. Nevertheless, illegal drug use is widely considered to be a significant problem in the indigenous population, and there is growing evidence of problematic use among other ethnic groups. The lack of access to treatment by these populations is of considerable concern. Various ethnic groups are also implicated in the importation and distribution of specific illegal drugs, although the clear demarcation between ethnic groups is declining as the multiculturalism of Australian society is increasingly reflected in its organized crime (National Crime Authority 2001).

In the Australian federal system, state and territory governments are responsible for drug policies. These can be influenced by the federal government via national drug policies and funding to the states and territories. In addition, the federal government is responsible for international treaties. Although cultural, policy, and trade influence shifted from the United Kingdom to the United States after World War II, Australia has developed its own pragmatic approach rather than adopting U.S. drug policies. A hallmark of Australian national drug policy is that it includes alcohol, tobacco, and psychoactive prescription drugs as well as illegal drugs, although we only discuss the last of these.

Prevalence of illicit drug use

The federal government conducts regular household surveys of representative samples of Australians, which generally provide reasonably accurate estimates of the use of cannabis, amphetamines, and hallucinogens but probably underestimate heroin and cocaine use. Results from the most recent household survey in 1998 (Australian Institute of Health and Welfare 1999) are presented in Figure 1.

Cannabis is the most widely used illicit drug, with 39 percent of those ages fourteen years and older using it at some time in their lives and 18

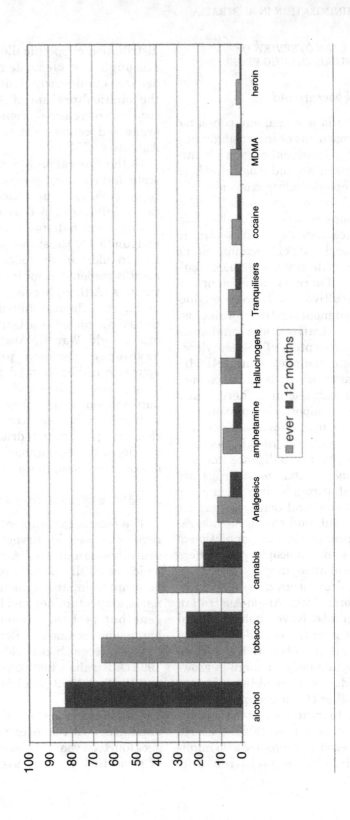

FIGURE 1
PREVALENCE OF ILLICIT DRUG USE AMONG AUSTRALIAN ADULTS

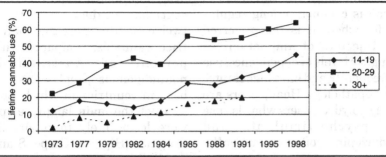

FIGURE 2
**LIFETIME PREVALENCE OF CANNABIS USE
AMONG AUSTRALIANS, 1973 TO 1998, BY AGE**

percent having done so in the past year. Cannabis users are more likely to be male, younger than thirty-five years of age, and unemployed than nonusers. Better-educated people are more likely to have tried cannabis but use it less often than less-educated persons. Younger users prefer to use a bong or pipe while older users prefer joints. In Australia, about 10 percent of people who ever try cannabis become daily users, and another 20 to 30 percent use weekly. Lifetime cannabis use increased between 1973 and 1998 (see Figure 2).

Around 2 percent of people older than fourteen have tried heroin at least once, and slightly more than 1 percent have used heroin five or more times in the past year. There were estimated to be 74,000 dependent heroin users in 1997-1998 (range = 67,000 to 92,000) (Hall et al. 2000): 6.9 per 1,000 adults ages fifteen to fifty-four years. Heroin use appears to have increased during the mid-1990s.

The typical dependent heroin user in cross-sectional surveys is around thirty years of age, with about twice as many men as women and most being unemployed. While there is recreational heroin use, it is the dependent heroin user who has the greatest impact on public health and public order. Recent studies have shown that the age of onset of heroin use is falling, with initiation occurring in the mid-teens, where previously it was around eighteen to nineteen years of age.

The majority of heroin users inject the drug, but recently there has been a diffusion of heroin smoking, particularly among Indo-Chinese populations in Australia, with many smokers making a transition to injecting. Many Australian heroin users injected amphetamines before heroin, and polydrug use is the norm, with many heroin users also dependent on alcohol, amphetamines, and benzodiazepines.

Amphetamine derivates have been used by 9 percent of Australian adults and by 21 percent of twenty- to twenty-nine-year-olds at some time in their lives. Males are more likely than females to have used amphetamines, typically in their mid- to late-teens, generally orally or intra-nasally rather than by injection.

Around 17 percent of those who had used amphetamines in the past year reported injecting. The transition to injecting is common among regular users for whom it is the preferred route. Injectors of amphetamines have higher levels of dependence, use more frequently, and have higher rates of psychopathology. Heavy users are typically polydrug users who also use other psychostimulants and benzodiazepines, often concurrently.

Lifetime use of the amphetamine analogue MDMA appears to have increased from 2 percent in 1995 to 5 percent in 1998, with 2 percent reporting use in the preceding twelve months. MDMA users usually are in their twenties, are well educated, and are more likely to be employed than users of other illicit drugs. Rates of use are only slightly higher among males than females. Most use is less than weekly, but the frequency of use may be increasing, as may bingeing.

Lifetime use of cocaine is at 3 to 4 percent of adults, with around 1 percent using in the preceding twelve months. Cocaine injection increased sharply in the late 1990s among injecting drug users in Sydney but has not yet increased in other states.

Lifetime use of LSD and other hallucinogens is estimated at around 10 percent, an increase on the 6 to 7 percent from earlier surveys. Rates of use in the past twelve months are around 3 percent, with most use occasional.

There are limited data on drug use among Australians from different cultural backgrounds. Illicit drug use among indigenous Australians appears to be high, with approximately 59 percent older than fourteen years having tried an illicit drug and almost a quarter (23 percent) having done so in the past twelve months. More than half have tried cannabis, compared with 39 percent of Australian-born nonindigenous people. Australians born in countries in which English was not the main language spoken were least likely to report illicit drug use (Higgins, Cooper-Stanbury, and Williams 2000).

Caution needs to be exercised when comparing drug use across different countries because of different methods of data collection. Even so, Australia seems to have higher rates of lifetime or recent cannabis use than the United States or Europe. Thirty-nine percent of Australians had ever used cannabis, and 18 percent had done so in the past twelve months, compared with 33 percent and 9 percent in the United States (Department of Health and Human Services 1999), 22 percent and 9 percent in the United Kingdom, and 18 percent and 5 percent in the Netherlands (European Monitoring Centre for Drugs and Drug Addiction 1999).

The prevalence of heroin dependence in Australia (7 per 1,000 adults ages fifteen to fifty-four, range = 5-8) (Hall et al. 2000) is comparable to that in the European Union (namely, 3 to 8 per 1,000) (European Monitoring Centre for Drugs and Drug Addiction 1999) and the same as the United Kingdom's (7 per 1,000, range = 3-11). It is a little higher than estimates for the United States (5 per 1,000, range = 4-7) (Kessler et al. 1994). Australia and the United Kingdom have higher lifetime use of amphetamines (9 percent each) than the United States and other European countries, which have rates of less than 5 percent. Australia also has the highest lifetime use of MDMA, at 5 percent, but a much lower rate of lifetime cocaine use (3 percent) than the United States (10 percent).

*Costs and harms associated
   with illicit drug use—
Distinctive Australian features*

The estimated costs of illicit drug abuse, including control costs and economic costs of premature loss of life, for 1992, were Australian$1.7 billion. The tangible costs, largely health service costs (in current prices) rose from Australian$908 million in 1988 to Australian$1,248 million in 1992, representing a 37 percent increase. These estimates do not include the costs of crime, ambulance services, welfare, absenteeism, and turnover of other drugs (Collins and Lapsley 1996). Collins and Lapsley (1996) estimated that law enforcement costs (up 41 percent from Australian$320 million in 1988 to Australian$450.6 million in 1992) accounted for more than one-third of total costs in both years, an increase of 23 percent in real terms. This amounts to around 0.4 percent of GDP.

Marks (1992) estimated that property crime losses as a result of illicit drug use cost Australia Australian$466 million in 1988 and that property crime accounted for 32 percent of total costs of law enforcement. A survey of two hundred heroin users in southwestern Sydney indicated that illegal activities, predominantly acquisitive property crime and the sale and distribution of illicit drugs, accounted for 82 percent of the sample's income in the week before the interview. From these data it was estimated that the total cost of heroin-related crime in Australia was between Australian$535 million and Australian$1.6 billion per annum.

Australia has two distinctive features associated with harms from illicit injecting drug use—high rates of death from heroin and other opioid-related overdose and low rates of HIV infection attributable to injecting drug use.

The number of fatal opioid overdoses rose from 6 in 1964 to 600 in 1997, a 55-fold increase in rate when adjusted for growth in population (Hall, Lynskey, and Degenhardt 1999). This increased again in 1998 to 738 deaths. Nonfatal opioid overdoses are extremely common, with recent studies reporting a lifetime rate of 67 percent among dependent heroin users (Darke, Ross, and Hall 1996). The typical overdose fatality is a single, unemployed, thirty-year-old man, who is a long-term dependent heroin user and who was not in treatment at the time of death. For both fatal and nonfatal overdoses, there is a strong association with the concomitant use of alcohol and benzodiazepines. In early 2001, Australia experienced a "heroin drought" and a sharp decrease in overdose deaths. For example, in Victoria, there were 214 deaths in the first seven months of 2000, but there were only 29 in 2001.

To date, Australia has averted an epidemic of HIV infection, both in the population at large and among injecting drug users. Approximately 8 percent of new HIV cases occur in injecting drug users, of whom slightly less than half are men with a history of male sexual contact. The prevalence of HIV infection among people attending needle and syringe programs in Australia has been estimated at less than 3 percent (MacDonald et al. 1997). This low rate of HIV infection among injecting drug users may reflect Australia's geographic isolation, its relatively low numbers of visitors and immigrants, and the early introduction of needle and syringe programs.

In contrast, 50 percent of injecting drug users are infected with hepatitis C. While the routes of transmission are the same as for HIV, hepatitis C seems to be more infectious but less lethal, although the liver disease it causes can be fatal. The rate of new hepatitis C infections among injecting drug users is estimated to be around 15 percent per year.

DISTINCTIVE FEATURES OF AUSTRALIAN DRUG POLICY

Since illicit drug use among young Australians was first observed in the larger Australian cities in the mid- to late 1960s (Manderson 1993), Australia has incrementally increased police powers and penalties relating to illicit drugs. Nonetheless, Australian society has shown a long-standing ambivalence about whether to adopt a moral or a therapeutic approach to illicit drug users. Australian states treat the use of cannabis, cocaine, heroin, and other illicit drugs as criminal offences, and property offences to fund illicit drug use

are common among prisoners. Government inquiries into drug use and ways of ameliorating its effects have been a feature of the Australian response to the problem. There were more than ten major inquiries between 1971 and 1991 and more inquiries since then.

Since the mid-1980s, Australia has evolved a set of policies based on its own experience and borrowing from experience in Europe and North America. The punitive and moralistic approach of the United States has been largely avoided, making it possible to discuss drug law reform without the personal attacks on the motives of critics seen in the United States. Australia has from time to time been influenced by overseas drug policies and programs, with policy entrepreneurs encouraging the adoption of seemingly plausible programs in the absence of a strong evidence base (e.g., drug courts and ultrarapid opiate detoxification using naltrexone).

Notwithstanding these exceptions and the martial rhetoric of "national campaigns," a "drug offensive," and "tough on drugs," public health concepts have had an effect on the national drug strategy, usually in combination with law enforcement and interdiction. The overarching aim of the 1986 National Campaign Against Drug Abuse was to "minimise the harmful effects of drugs on Australian society" (Blewett 1987, 2). This was undertaken through education and information provision, a significant expansion of treatment, and collection of national data on drug use and drug-related harm. In treatment there was emphasis on early intervention in primary health care settings, specialist drug-specific settings, and evaluation. There was new funding for research with the establishment of two national research centers and, later, a third national center for education and training.

Although harm minimization has been the basis of Australia's policy for more than two decades, its meaning is not universally agreed on. Australia's harm minimization approach was exemplified by the response to the burgeoning international HIV epidemic in the early 1980s. This involved frank public education campaigns and the rapid introduction of needle and syringe exchange programs. Other measures included the diversion of drug offenders into treatment, expansion of methadone maintenance and drug-free treatment programs, and the encouragement of police officers to use their discretion in not enforcing laws against the possession of injecting equipment.

Australia has also been fortunate in that the policy of harm minimization has, until recently, enjoyed bipartisan political support at federal and state levels. It may be that bipartisanship was easier in Australia than in the United States because of the tighter control that political parties exercise over politicians in Australia. This minimizes the opportunity for politicians to pursue populist policies on illicit drug use.

A noteworthy success of the Australian drug strategy has been intersectoral collaboration between health and law enforcement. There are variations in how local police carry out their duties throughout Australia, but there is a growing awareness that policing can increase as well as decrease harms. In the past few years, this has prompted a move toward policing that might be described as moderating or regulating the drug marketplace. While saturation and drug blitz operations still occur, there is recognition that different strategies are appropriate for different locations, depending on the type of drug market and the population mix. It is also noteworthy that an open street drug-trading scene is a relatively recent phenomenon in this country. Its appearance has significantly increased community concern about safety, public nuisance, and public amenity in specific areas in our major cities. This, in turn, has provided the rationale for a formally evaluated trial, starting in 2001, of a medically supervised injecting place in one of the major areas of drug trading in Sydney.

Bipartisan support for harm minimization weakened after 1997. An important trigger was the veto by the prime minister and cabinet of a proposed trial of heroin prescribing (see below) that had been approved by a majority of state, territory, and federal health and law enforcement ministers. Loss of bipartisanship also blocked trials of supervised injecting places in Victoria and the Australian Capital Territory.

After blocking the heroin trial, the federal government allocated more than Australian$500 million to education, treatment, and law enforcement to address the high rates of opioid overdose deaths and crime that were highlighted in the debate about a heroin trial. In addition, Prime Minister John Howard attempted to reduce the role of harm reduction in state drug policies by making critical statements about state and territory policies and by directly giving federal funds to treatment services, thereby bypassing state and territory governments. He also appointed a new council, the Australian National Council on Drugs, to advise him and selected as its chair someone who publicly opposed a heroin trial and was historically antagonistic to harm minimization programs.

There was a subsequent debate about whether harm minimization should be the goal of national drug policy. The term survived in a compromise national policy document as referring to policies and programs that aimed at "reducing drug-related harm" and as a term that "encompasses a wide range of approaches, including abstinence-oriented strategies." It was taken as "preventing anticipated harm as well as reducing actual harm" and regarded as being "consistent with a comprehensive approach to drug-related harm, involving a balance between demand reduction, supply reduction and harm reduction"(Ministerial Council on Drug Strategy 1998). Current national policy uses the rhetoric of "tough on drugs" to cover a strong budgetary emphasis on law enforcement and interdiction together with increased funding for abstinence-oriented treatment and programs that aim to reduce imprisonment by diverting drug users into treatment and rehabilitation.

Other aspects of Australia's drug policy that are noteworthy include the following:

- a critical mass of research and policy expertise despite the small population;
- a mixture of government and nongovernment programs in prevention and treatment;
- slow narrowing of a twenty-year separation between drug dependence and mental health, in both treatment and prevention;
- a powerful and concentrated media, which "has been a ... distorting mirror ... of society's attitude toward drug use, . . . giving warped and false images to the public at large" (Fox and Mathews 1992, 173)—the expansion of talk-back radio has magnified this distortion;
- government-funded drug user groups, which provide peer services, undertake advocacy, and undertake a range of projects; and
- services designed to support families of drug users.

TWO CASE STUDIES— CANNABIS AND HEROIN

We illustrate Australia's approach by using policies toward cannabis and heroin. In the case of cannabis, we describe the impact of legislation that punishes simple cannabis offences by payment of a fine (so-called expiation). Most of the evidence comes from the state of South Australia, where this legislation was introduced in 1986. Such legislation also exists in the Australian Capital Territory (1992) and the Northern Territory (1997). For heroin, we examine the changing role of treatment with opioid drugs that have a similar mechanism of action to heroin, with a particular focus on the mainstay of treatment, methadone maintenance. We also examine an unsuccessful attempt to trial heroin maintenance and recent trials of the agonist LAAM, the partial agonist buprenorphine, and the antagonist (heroin-blocking drug) naltrexone.

Cannabis

In 1979, the South Australian Royal Commission into the Non-Medical Use of Drugs recommended that minor cannabis use not be treated as a criminal offence. After an intense and lengthy community debate, the South Australian Cannabis Expiation Notice (CEN) system was introduced in 1987. Under this system, police issue an expiation notice for minor cannabis offences, that is, possession of up to one hundred grams of cannabis, possession of twenty grams of cannabis resin or equipment for consuming cannabis, or cultivation of a specified (low) number of cannabis plants. If the expiation fee (ranging from Australian$50 to Australian$150) is paid within thirty to sixty days, criminal proceedings are avoided, and no offence is recorded. Failure to pay leads to criminal proceedings and often results in a criminal conviction.

The experience of some U.S. states that had adopted a similar approach inspired the introduction of the South Australian scheme. While the U.S. influence in that state was indirect and supportive of the change, when the Australian Capital Territory proposed a similar change in the early 1990s, the U.S. Information Service brought to Australia Dr.

Gabriel Nahas, who campaigned for a more punitive approach to cannabis by holding public meetings, making media statements, and publishing an article in the *Medical Journal of Australia* on the toxicity of marijuana (Nahas and Latour 1992).

There were no planned evaluations of the legislative changes, but there have been a number of post facto analyses of the impact of the South Australian system. Survey data on drug use have not found an increase in cannabis use attributable to the CEN scheme. In addition, neither the CEN scheme nor the more usual punitive approach have any deterrent effect on continuing use, as revealed by interviews with minor cannabis offenders in South Australia and Western Australia, most of whom reported that they would not stop using even if they were caught again.

The CEN scheme has led to an increase in the number of minor cannabis offences detected from around 6,000 in 1987-1988 to approximately 17,000 in 1993-1994 and later years (Christie 1999). This net widening was not due to changes in patterns of cannabis use. It reflected the ease with which police can issue expiation notices and a move away from police giving informal cautions to recording all minor offences.

Since the inception of the CEN scheme, the rate of payment of expiation fees has remained at around 50 percent. The majority who do not pay are convicted and receive fines similar to the original expiation fees, plus court fees. As significant numbers of those issued a summons plead guilty in writing rather than appearing in person, the burden on the court system has been reduced.

A survey of law enforcement and criminal justice personnel found strong support for the CEN scheme. It was perceived to be cost efficient, to be convenient for police officers, and to lessen the negative social impacts of a conviction. Specialist drug enforcement personnel voiced a concern about the (then) limit of ten cannabis plants in cultivation that they believed criminal groups were exploiting by combining the output of multiple plots of ten plants. As a consequence, the expiable number of plants was reduced to three, and the South Australian government is considering a further reduction to one plant and removing hydroponically grown cannabis from expiable offences.

An economic evaluation of the scheme (Brooks et al. 1999) estimated the total cost (not including police time in detecting the offence) at Australian$1.2 million in 1995-1996 while revenue from fees and fines was Australian$1.7 million. The cost-effectiveness would be greater if the proportion of offenders who paid the initial fines was increased.

The introduction of a CEN scheme seems to have confused the general population about the legal status of cannabis use. In 1993, for example, 34 percent of South Australians and 43 percent of residents of the Australian Capital Territory mistakenly believed that it was legal to possess cannabis for personal use, compared with less than 10 percent of respondents in most other parts of Australia (Bowman and Sanson-Fisher

1994). A more recent evaluation showed similar results.

It is doubtful that the CEN scheme had any impact on the attitudes of the general population toward cannabis use. The South Australian community seems to be fairly tolerant of personal cannabis use, but so is the rest of Australia because more than 70 percent of the Australian public believe that civil, rather than criminal, penalties should apply to minor cannabis offences (Bowman and Sanson-Fisher 1994). This support is strongly linked to personal or vicarious (through friends) experience with cannabis.

Apart from the one state and two territories that have legislated prohibition with civil penalties, the other states of Australia are diverting offenders to education and treatment while retaining criminal penalties. The underlying philosophies have been different in different states. For example, in Victoria, the aim is to provide support, information, and potential referral to other services. In Western Australia, on the other hand, the program is a deliberate effort within a tough-on-drugs philosophy to "capture" as many early cannabis users as possible to receive compulsory education.

Heroin

Alcohol treatment programs began to see heroin-dependent people in very small numbers in the early 1970s, when injecting heroin first became evident in Australia. Treatment included withdrawal, treatment of concurrent illness, variable periods of supportive counseling, and occasionally residential rehabilitation.

Methadone was introduced into Australia in 1970 to provide a legal and controlled supply of an orally administered opioid drug that only had to be taken once a day because its long duration of action eliminated opiate withdrawal symptoms for twenty-four to thirty-six hours. After initial enthusiasm for methadone treatment, the number of places in the two most populous states, New South Wales and Victoria, contracted in the late 1970s and early 1980s. Increasing demand for places and fears of an epidemic of HIV/AIDS among injecting drug users led to an increase in treatment places in the mid-1980s after methadone treatment was endorsed by a national drug summit in 1985. The number of people in methadone treatment rose from 2,203 in February 1985 to 26,677 in 1999 (Hall et al. 2000). The proportion of regular heroin users enrolled in methadone treatment was estimated to be around 17 percent in 1987, rising to 31 percent in 1997.

The expansion of methadone maintenance treatment was accomplished in part by growth in the private sector from 1,745 to 8,449 places while numbers in public programs increased from 2,701 in June 1987 to 6,541 in June 1994. Private programs are run by general practitioners or psychiatrists, who are licensed by the state or territory government to prescribe methadone for opioid dependence. Methadone is dispensed either at the private clinic or through community pharmacies. Medical services and pathology are funded federally, and dispensing costs of Australian$40 to Australian$50 per week are borne by the client. Public programs are now also increasingly charging clients. For those who derive their income from social welfare, which is a large proportion of clients, the fees are a substantial part of their income. It has been claimed that this money may be raised by selling take-away methadone doses or by property crime.

In the 1990s, clients were no longer expelled from methadone treatment for continued heroin use in recognition of the benefits of keeping people in treatment. There have been fluctuations in policies on take-away doses of methadone: more liberal policies in the early 1990s were introduced to enable clients to live more normal lives; more restrictive policies in the later 1990s were motivated by concerns about diversion and injection of methadone syrup and by some methadone-linked deaths.

Despite the scale of methadone maintenance treatment in Australia, there is political ambivalence about whether it should be provided. One consequence of this ambivalence is that many programs have provided what research indicates is substandard treatment. Entry to treatment was made difficult for fear of creating iatrogenic dependence, and patients received low doses of methadone for fear of prolonging dependence. Many programs also encouraged their patients to achieve abstinence within a year or two, with staff interpreting their inability to do so as evidence of the failure of methadone maintenance treatment. A book-length review by Ward, Mattick, and Hall (1992) played a role in changing poor procedures by reinforcing the evidence base for treatment practice.

In 1991, a feasibility study began looking into providing heroin as an adjunct treatment for heroin dependence, and a controlled trial was recommended in 1995 (Bammer and Douglas 1996). After a period of intense debate, the trial was blocked by the federal government, but a trial continues to be advocated by eminent individuals and organizations.

There has been interest in other pharmacotherapies for opioid dependence, but the necessary convergence of political, drug company, treatment provider, research, and community support did not exist until the late 1990s when national trials of buprenorphine, LAAM, and naltrexone led to burprenorphine (2001) and naltrexone (1999) being registered for the treatment of opioid dependence. The incorporation of these drugs into treatment programs may have been facilitated by the blocking of the heroin trial.

Recent years have also seen a significant expansion of services specifically for young people. There are also diversion programs in the legal process at arrest, presentencing, and suspended sentencing; the provision of active treatment in jail; transition programs for those leaving jail and access to treatment on exit; and the provision of methadone treatment in some prisons. Some of these are still experimental, some have broad support, and others are more controversial, but public debate has allowed increasing diversity of treatment.

CONCLUSION

Australia now faces a number of challenges in its drug policy. These include the loss of bipartisan support and an increasingly polarized debate, the increasing use of cocaine, and unless the heroin drought proves lasting, a very high overdose death rate. Nevertheless, the positive aspects of Australia's drug policy remain in place, innovations can still find support, and an independent humane pragmatism continues to be the overarching approach.

References

For reasons of space, only the minimum references are presented. A full list is available from the authors.

Australian Institute of Health and Welfare. 1999. *1998 National Drug Strategy Household Survey: First results.* Drug Statistics Series cat. no. PHE 15. Canberra: Australian Institute of Health and Welfare.

Bammer, G., and R. M. Douglas. 1996. The ACT heroin trial proposal: An overview. *Medical Journal of Australia* 164:690-92.

Blewett, N. 1987. *NCADA: Assumptions, arguments and aspirations.* National Campaign against Drug Abuse Monograph Series no. 1. Canberra: Australian Government.

Bowman, J., and R. Sanson-Fisher. 1994. *Public perceptions of cannabis legislation.* National Drug Strategy Monograph Series no. 28. Canberra: Australian Government.

Brooks, A., C. Stothard, J. Moss, P. Christie, and R. Ali. 1999. *Costs associated with the operation of the Cannabis Expiation Notice scheme in South Australia.* DASC Monograph no. 5.

Adelaide, Australia: Drug & Alcohol Services Council.

Christie, P. 1999. *Cannabis offences under the Cannabis Expiation Notice scheme in South Australia*. National Drug Strategy Monograph Series no. 35. Canberra: Australian Government.

Collins, D., and H. Lapsley. 1996. *The social costs of drug abuse in Australia in 1988 and 1992*. Canberra: Australian Government.

Darke, S., J. Ross, and W. Hall. 1996. Overdose among heroin users in Sydney, Australia: I. Prevalence and correlates of non-fatal overdose. *Addiction* 91:405-11.

Department of Health and Human Services. Substance Abuse and Mental Health Services Administration. 1999. *Summary of findings from the 1998 National Household Survey on Drug Abuse*. National Household Survey on Drug Abuse Series no. H-10. Rockville, MD: Department of Health and Human Services.

European Monitoring Center for Drugs and Drug Addiction. 1999. *Extended annual report on the state of the drugs problem in the European Union*. Luxembourg,: Office for Official Publications of the European Communities.

Fox, R., and I. Mathews. 1992. *Drugs policy: Fact, fiction and the future*. Sydney, Australia: Federation Press.

Hall, W., M. Lynskey, and L. Degenhardt. 1999. *Heroin use in Australia: Its impact on public health and public order*. NDARC Monograph no. 42. Sydney, Australia: University of New South Wales.

Hall, W., J. Ross, M. Lynskey, M. Law, and L. Degenhardt. 2000. How many dependent heroin users are there in Australia? *Medical Journal of Australia* 173:528-31.

Higgins, K., M. Cooper-Stanbury, and P. Williams. 2000. *Statistics on drug use in Australia 1998*. Drug Statistics Series cat. no. PHE 16. Canberra: Australian Institute of Health and Welfare.

Kessler, R. C., K. A. McGonagh, S. Zhao, C. B. Nelson, M. Hughes, S. Eshelman, U. Wittchen, and K. S. Kendler. 1994. Lifetime and 12-month prevalence of DSM-III-R psychiatric disorders in the United States. *Archives of General Psychiatry* 51:8-19.

MacDonald, M., A. Wodak, R. Ali, N. Crofts, P. Cunningham, K. Dolan, M. Kelaher, W. Loxley, I. Van Beek, and J. Kaldor. 1997. HIV prevalence and risk behaviours in needle exchange attenders: A national study. *Medical Journal of Australia* 166:237-40.

Manderson, D. 1993. *From Mr Sin to Mr Big: A history of Australian drug laws*. Melbourne, Australia: Oxford University Press.

Marks, R. E. 1992. Costs of illegal drug use. In *The consequences of alcohol and drug use: Implications for policy*, NDARC Monograph no. 15, edited by W. Swift. Sydney, Australia: University of New South Wales.

Ministerial Council on Drug Strategy. 1998. *National drug strategic framework, 1998-99 to 2002-03: Building partnerships—A strategy to reduce the harm caused by drugs in our community*. Canberra: Commonwealth of Australia.

Nahas, G., and C. Latour. 1992. The human toxicity of marijuana. *Medical Journal of Australia* 156:495-97.

National Crime Authority. 2001. *Organised crime in Australia: NCA commentary 2001*. Sydney, Australia: National Crime Authority.

Ward, J., R. Mattick, and W. Hall. 1992. *Key issues in methadone maintenance*. Sydney, Australia: University of New South Wales Press.

Science, Ideology, and
Needle Exchange Programs

By MARTIN T. SCHECHTER

ABSTRACT: Needle exchange programs (NEPs) to prevent HIV transmission among injection drug users are accepted in many countries but remain at the center of heated debate in the United States. In 1997, the author published a study of injection drug users in Vancouver showing an explosive outbreak of HIV. An incidental finding was higher HIV rates among frequent attendees of the local NEP. While this was expected because NEPs attract users at highest risk, opponents of needle exchange applied an unsupportable causal interpretation to this finding. If frequent NEP attendees had higher HIV rates, so the interpretation went, NEPs must be responsible for promoting the spread of HIV. Despite the author's admonitions against this misinterpretation of the data, it was used as part of a successful campaign to oppose U.S. federal funding of needle exchange. Regrettably, biased or even misleading interpretations often occur in the volatile interface of imperfect science and ideological debate.

Martin T. Schechter is a professor and the head of the Department of Health Care and Epidemiology in the Faculty of Medicine at the University of British Columbia. He completed his Ph.D. in mathematics at the Polytechnic Institute of New York, his M.D. at McMaster University, and his master's degree in epidemiology at the University of Toronto. He is the Canada Research Chair in HIV/AIDS and Urban Population Health and the director of epidemiology at the B.C. Centre for Excellence in HIV/AIDS.

NOTE: Support for this research was provided by National Institute on Drug Abuse and the Canadian Institutes of Health Research. Dr. Schechter holds a tier I Canada Research Chair in HIV/AIDS and Urban Population Health.

NEEDLE exchange programs (NEPs) have become a cornerstone for prevention of blood-borne pathogens among injection drug users (IDUs) in most developed countries and a growing number of developing countries. In the United States, Kaplan, Khoshnood, and Heimer (1994) demonstrated that NEP use in New Haven was associated with a reduction in HIV incidence. Likewise, Hagan and colleagues (1995) reported that the nonuse of NEPs was associated with an elevated risk for hepatitis B and C infection among IDUs in Tacoma. Studies in Amsterdam, Sydney, Glasgow, London, and Sweden found that HIV incidence and syringe sharing behavior either remained low or declined significantly over time following NEP introduction (Van Ameijden, Van Den Hoek, and Coutinho 1994; Hunter, Donoghoe, Stimson, et al. 1995; Ljungberg, Christensson, Tunving, et al. 1991). However, decreases in HIV incidence could not be directly attributed to NEP use. In a global survey of eighty-one cities with available data on IDUs, Hurley, Jolley, and Kaldor (1997) estimated HIV prevalence decreased an average of 5.8 percent per year in twenty-nine cities with established NEPs but increased an average of 5.9 percent per year in fifty-one cities without such programs. However, despite research from North America (Hurley, Jolley, and Kaldor 1997) and Europe (Stimson 1995; Gruer, Cameron, and Elliott 1993) that demonstrates the positive benefits of NEPs, they remain highly controversial, particularly in the United States.

THE SETTING

The downtown east side of Vancouver is approximately half a square mile of pawn shops, secondhand stores, single room apartment/hotels, the homeless, sex workers, a noticeable police presence, and families trying to raise children in a hostile environment. It has been home to one of the largest concentrations of illicit drug users in Canada for many decades (Canadian Government Commission 1972). To combat the spread of infectious diseases among Vancouver's IDUs, a NEP was established in Vancouver's downtown east side in 1988. This was the first NEP in Canada and one of the earliest on the continent. Vancouver's NEP has reportedly maintained its status as the largest in North America (Canadian HIV AIDS Legal Network 1999), exchanging more than 2 million needles per year by 1996 and 3 million by 1999.

During 1996-1997, my research team documented an explosive outbreak of HIV among IDUs in Vancouver's downtown east side. In this period, we reported that the prevalence of HIV infection among drug users was 23 percent and, more important, that the annual rate of new cases had reached as high as 18 percent per year, an alarmingly high incidence rate (Strathdee et al. 1997). In the latter report, which was purposefully titled "Needle Exchange Is Not Enough: Lessons from the Vancouver Injection User Study," we argued that the protective effects of even a large-volume NEP could be overwhelmed if the NEP were operating in the absence of adequate complementary services such as detoxification and accessible addiction treatment.

THE CONTEXT

At the time of publication of this article, a ban on the use of federal funds for NEPs is in place in the United States. Despite a 1991 U.S. Government Accounting Office study that concluded that NEPs "hold some promise as an AIDS prevention strategy," Congress had passed legislation in 1992 prohibiting the use of federal funds to support NEPs until the surgeon general could certify that they did not encourage drug use and were effective in reducing the spread of HIV. By 1997, several U.S. government–sponsored reports had reached these two conclusions. For example, in March 1997, the National Institutes of Health published the *Consensus Development Statement on Interventions to Prevent HIV Risk Behaviors* that concluded NEPs "show a reduction in risk behaviors as high as 80% in injecting drug users, with estimates of a 30% or greater reduction of HIV" (p. 5). In February 1997, then secretary of Health and Human Services Shalala (Department of Health and Human Services 1998) reported to Congress that a review of scientific studies indicated that NEPs "can be an effective component of a comprehensive strategy to prevent HIV and other blood borne infectious diseases in communities that choose to include them" (p. 1). Nevertheless, debate about the effectiveness of NEPs raged between proponents and

opponents throughout 1997 in anticipation of a decision by the U.S. administration as to whether to lift the ban on federal funding, scheduled for the spring of 1998.

THE INCRIMINATING EVIDENCE

In our article published in July 1997 (Strathdee et al. 1997), we presented a substantial amount of data from our prospective study of more than 1,000 IDUs in Vancouver. However, one specific finding within the article was to receive the lion's share of the attention. The result in question was that among frequent attendees of the Vancouver NEP (i.e., drug users who visited the NEP once or more per week), the prevalence of HIV infection was observed to be approximately 32 percent, whereas it was 14 percent among less frequent attendees. To us, this was not a surprising finding.

Unfortunately, there are ways to misinterpret data such as these. The simplest approach is as follows: if a greater proportion of those who visit the NEP frequently have HIV than those who visit less frequently, then the NEP must be responsible for causing HIV infection among its attendees. Under the circumstances, NEP should be considered harmful. In epidemiology, we would refer to this as a causal association. This interpretation is simple, direct, and straightforward. However, in this instance, it is also incorrect as we will see later. But the simple cause and effect interpretation proved particularly appealing to those in search of evidence detrimental to NEPs.

THE POLITICAL INTERPRETATION

On 11 September 1997, Representative Dennis Hastert proposed an amendment to a yearly appropriations act that would prohibit the use of federal funds for NEPs indefinitely. During debate in the House of Representatives in September 1997, he stated, "What the Vancouver studies have shown is that intravenous drug users who use the needle exchange have a greater chance of becoming HIV positive than intravenous drug users who do not use the needle exchange" (Departments of Labor, Health and Human Services, and Education et al.; H7218).

On 21 April 1998, Senator Paul Coverdell, along with Senators Ashcroft and Brownback, introduced the Needle Exchange Programs Prohibition Act of 1998, a bill to prohibit the use of federal funds to carry out or support programs for the distribution of sterile hypodermic needles or syringes to illegal drug users. During introduction of the bill, Senator Coverdell stated that in Vancouver, "HIV infections were higher among users of free needles than those without access to them" (Congressional Record 1998).

A congressional press conference was held on 22 April 1998 by Representatives Gingrich, Hastert, Delay, and Wicker to discuss a House bill banning use of federal funds for NEPs. At that time, Representative Hastert stated, "If you look at . . . Vancouver, for instance, you'll find that when you start to hand out free needles, HIV incidence goes up. . . . The science doesn't prove [NEP is effective] and I have a copy of the Vancouver study that shows that." Representative Wicker said that in Vancouver, "addicts receiving free needles were becoming HIV positive at twice the rate of others not in the program."

Quite obviously then, these political leaders opted for the causal interpretation. The blame for the fact that the frequent NEP attendees had higher rates of HIV than the less frequent attendees was laid clearly at the door of the NEP. Somehow the NEP must have been responsible for these higher rates, which would certainly be grounds to withdraw support for such programs.

EPIDEMIOLOGIC CONFOUNDING

Perhaps the simplest way to illustrate the error in logic is with some analogies. In the example of NEPs and HIV, the logical argument goes something like this: frequent attendees of the NEP have higher HIV prevalence rates than less frequent attendees. Therefore, the NEP must be responsible in some way for increased spread of HIV among its users. Therefore, NEPs should be closed.

Now consider the following observation. People who attend the opera have greater wealth than people who do not attend. Following the same causal interpretation, one might conclude that the opera is somehow responsible for increasing the wealth of people who attend it. A policy recommendation that might follow from this would be to encourage people to attend the opera as a way of increasing their wealth.

What about the situation in hospitals? It is clearly the case that people who are admitted to hospitals have higher death rates than people who are not admitted. Should one conclude that hospitals are responsible for killing the patients they admit? If so, the logical policy recommendation would be to close hospitals down.

A moment's reflection should bring the misinterpretation into clear relief. The reason people who are admitted to hospitals have higher death rates than people not admitted is that people requiring hospital admission are inherently sicker. Indeed, that is presumably the reason they are in the hospital. The hospital is not responsible for the higher death rates; they occur because the hospital is coping with a population in far worse health than those who remain out in the community.

Is the opera responsible for increasing the wealth of its patrons? Not likely. It is simply that those individuals who choose to attend (or can afford to attend) the opera have greater wealth than those who choose not to (or cannot) attend.

Is the NEP in Vancouver responsible for the higher prevalence rates of HIV among its frequent attendees? Or is it simply the case that those IDUs who most use the services of the NEP are the very ones whose behaviors put them at greater risk of contracting HIV?

To answer this, we subsequently conducted a comparison of the HIV behavioral risk factors in frequent versus infrequent NEP attendees within our study. And as expected, we found very different risk profiles in the two groups. With regard to virtually every risk factor we know of that puts IDUs in our study at higher risk for contracting HIV, the frequent attendees had greater evidence of each. Specifically, when compared to infrequent attendees of the NEP, frequent attendees were younger, more likely to have poor housing situations, more likely to inject in so-called shooting galleries, more likely to inject cocaine on a daily basis, more likely to be involved in prostitution, more likely to have been incarcerated in the prior six months, and finally, less likely to be in methadone treatment for addiction (Schechter et al. 1999). Is it any wonder that they have higher rates of HIV than infrequent attendees? In fact, we went on to show that the excess in HIV rates among frequent attendees was precisely what one would expect based on their higher risk profiles.

As mentioned earlier, we were not at all surprised by our original finding of higher HIV rates among frequent NEP attendees. We understood the potential for epidemiologic confounding and had expected that frequent attendees would be those who were at highest risk of HIV. This should also not have been a mystery to readers of the 1997 article that first presented these controversial data (Strathdee et al. 1997). For we had warned readers very clearly about the potential for misinterpretation. Specifically, we had written in the very same article back in 1997 that the "fact that frequent NEP attendance was associated with HIV prevalence should not be interpreted as causal . . . NEPs attract higher risk injection drug users . . . and could thus be associated with HIV infection" (Strathdee et al. 1997; F64). Regrettably, as is clear from the above political statements, this warning was ignored.

MEDIA MISINTERPRETATION

Concerned about the misinterpretation's being applied to this research and that of Dr. Julie Bruneau, a colleague who had conducted a similar study in Montreal, Dr. Bruneau and I tried to set the record straight. In early April 1998, we faxed a 750-word opinion editorial to the *New York Times*. After substantial editing by the *Times*, a 380-word editorial appeared on 8 April 1998 (Bruneau and Schechter 1998). In it, Dr. Bruneau and I wrote,

In a letter to Congress, Barry McCaffrey, who is in charge of national drug policy, cited two Canadian studies to show that needle-exchange plans have failed to reduce the spread of HIV, the virus that causes AIDS, and may even have worsened the problem. Congressional leaders have cited these studies to make the same argument. As the authors of the Canadian studies, we must point out that these officials have misinterpreted our research. True, we found that addicts who took part in needle exchange programs in Vancouver and Montreal had higher HIV infection rates than addicts who did not. That's not surprising. Because these programs are in inner-city neighborhoods, they serve users who are at greatest risk of infection. Those who didn't accept free needles often didn't need them since they could afford to buy syringes in drug stores. They also were less likely to engage in the riskiest activities. (P. A31)

This opinion piece appeared several weeks before the statements of Senator Coverdell and Representatives Hastert and Wicker, cited above, but does not appear to have convinced them to reinterpret our scientific findings.

Two weeks later, the *New York Times* published a response written by Dr. James L. Curtis (1998), which, curiously, was allowed to run several hundred words longer than our original piece to which it responded. In it, Dr. Curtis wrote, "studies in Montreal and Vancouver . . . found that those addicts who took part in needle exchanges were two to three times more likely to become infected with HIV than those who did not participate" (p. A28). At this point, it appears that this was picked up by the wire services, and this same quote appeared in the *Seattle Post-Intelligencer*, the *Arizona Republic*, and the *Houston Chronicle*, among others.

THE FINAL STRAW

All through this period during March and April 1998, the Clinton administration was in the throes of a debate concerning whether to lift the ban on the federal funding of NEPs. Reportedly, Sandra Thurman, then White House director of AIDS policy, and the Presidential Council on HIV/AIDS both favored federal funding of NEPs, while Barry McCaffrey, the director of the Office of National Drug Control Policy, opposed it (Wren 1998).

In March of 1998, General McCaffrey dispatched a site visit team to Vancouver to investigate the situation in our setting. The two visitors, David Des Roches and Hoover Adger, spent several hours with our research team going over the findings of our study. During that meeting, we had the opportunity to present our data and, more important, to demonstrate to them in no uncertain terms that epidemiologic confounding had been responsible for the apparent association between frequent NEP attendance and HIV rates. We demonstrated for them that the frequent attendees had much riskier profiles than less frequent attendees (as outlined above), and that higher HIV rates were to be expected.

In their subsequent report to General McCaffrey (Des Roches 1998), the visitors wrote, "The HIV rates among participants in the NEP is higher than the HIV rate among injecting drug users who do not participate" (p. 2). There was no mention whatsoever of alternative explanations for this finding.

On Monday, 20 April 1998, the administration announced that it would not lift the ban on the federal funding of NEPs.

References

Bruneau, J., and M. T. Schechter. 1998. The politics of needles and AIDS. *New York Times*, 8 April, A31.

Canadian Government Commission of Inquiry into the Non-Medical Use of Drugs. 1972. Ottawa, Canada: Information Canada.

Canadian HIV AIDS Legal Network. 1999. *Injection drug use and HIV/AIDS: Legal and ethical issues.* Health Canada.

Congressional Record. 1998. 21 April. Senate pp. S3356-S3361.

Curtis J. L. 1998. Clean but not safe. *New York Times*, 22 April, A28.

Department of Health and Human Services. 1998. Research shows needle exchange programs reduce HIV infections without increasing drug use. Press release from HHS Press Office, 20 April. Retrieved from http://www.hhs.gov/news/press/1998pres/980420a.html.

Departments of Labor, Health and Human Services, and Education, and Related Agencies Appropriations Act, 1998. House of Representatives 11 September 1997:H7218.

Des Roches, D. B. 1998. Office of National Drug Control Policy (ONDCP), office memo to the director (Barry McCaffrey), ONDCP. Summation of field report based on site visit to Vancouver by Des Roches and Dr. Hoover Adger, deputy director, ONDCP. 6 April. Mimeographed.

Gruer, L., J. Cameron, and L. Elliott. 1993. Building a city wide service for exchanging needles and syringes. *British Medical Journal* 306:1394-97.

Hagan, H., D. C. DesJarlais, S. R. Friedman, D. Purchase, and M. J. Alter. 1995. Reduced risk of hepatitis B and hepatitis C among injection drug users in the Tacoma Syringe Exchange Program. *American Journal of Public Health* 85:1531-37.

Hunter G. M., M. C. Donoghoe, G. V. Stimson, et al. 1995. Changes in the injection risk behaviour of injecting drug users in London 1990-1993. *AIDS* 9:493-501.

Hurley S. F., D. J. Jolley, and J. M. Kaldor. 1997. Effectiveness of needle-exchange programmes for prevention of HIV infection. *Lancet* 349:1797-1800.

"Interventions to prevent HIV risk behaviors." 1997. *HIH Consensus Statement Online* 15(2): 1-41

Kaplan E. H., K. Khoshnood, and R. Heimer. 1994. A decline in HIV-infected needles returned to New Haven's needle exchange program: Client shift or needle exchange? *American Journal of Public Health* 84:1991-94.

Ljungberg, B., B. Christensson, K. Tunving, et al. 1991. HIV prevention among injecting drug users: Three years of experience from a syringe exchange program in Sweden. *Journal of AIDS* 4 (9): 890-95.

Schechter M. T., S. A. Strathdee, P. G. Cornelisse, K. J. Craib, S. Currie, D. M. Patrick, M. L. Rekart, and M. V. O'Shaughnessy. 1999. Do needle exchange programmes increase the spread of HIV among injection drug users? An investigation of the Vancouver outbreak. *AIDS* 13:F45-51.

Stimson, G. V. 1995. AIDS and injecting drug use in the United Kingdom, 1987-1993: The policy response and the prevention of the epidemic. *Social Science & Medicine* 41:699-716.

Strathdee, S. A., D. M. Patrick, S. L. Currie, P. G. Cornelisse, M. L. Rekart, J. S. Montaner, M. T. Schechter, and M. V. O'Shaughnessy. 1997. Needle exchange is not enough: Lessons from the Vancouver injecting drug use study. *AIDS* 11:F59-65.

U.S. General Accounting Office. March 1993. *Needle exchange programs: Research suggests promise as an AIDS prevention strategy.*

Van Ameijden, E.J.C., J.A.R. Van Den Hoek, and R. A. Coutinho. 1994. Injecting risk behaviour among drug users in Amsterdam, 1986 to 1992, and its relationship to AIDS prevention programs. *American Journal of Public Health* 84:275-81.

Wren, C. S. 1998. White House drug and AIDS advisers differ on needle exchange. *New York Times*, 23 March.

ANNALS, *AAPSS*, **582**, July 2002

Illegal Drugs in Colombia:
From Illegal Economic
Boom to Social Crisis

By FRANCISCO E. THOUMI

ABSTRACT: During the past thirty years, the illegal drug industry has marked Colombia's development. In no other country has the illegal drug industry had such dramatic social, political, and economic effects. This short article provides a synthesis of the development of the marijuana, coca-cocaine, and poppy-opium-heroin illegal industries. It studies the development of the drug cartels and marketing networks and the participation of guerrillas and paramilitary forces in the industry. The size of the illegal industry and its economic effects are also surveyed and its effects on the political system analyzed. The article ends with a discussion of the evolution of government policies and social attitudes toward the industry. The article shows that in the early years, the illegal industry was perceived by many as positive, how it evolved so that today it provides substantial funding for the country's ambiguous war, and that it is one of the main obstacles to peace.

Francisco E. Thoumi is a visiting scholar at the Latin American and Caribbean Center, Florida International University. He is a former research coordinator of the Office of Drug Control and Crime Prevention of the United Nations and a former fellow at the Woodrow Wilson Center for International Studies. He is the author of Political Economy and Illegal Drugs in Colombia *(1995, Lynne Rienner) and the forthcoming* Illegal Drugs Economy and Society in the Andes.

NOTE: The author thanks Peter Reuter for his comments on an earlier draft and exonerates him of any responsibility for the contents of this article.

AT the turn of the twenty-first century, Colombian society is in a profound crisis in which illegal drugs play a very complex and important role. Colombia is the only country in the world where the three main plant-based illegal drugs are produced in significant amounts. Colombians are involved in illegal drug production, international smuggling, and marketing. In the 1980s, Colombia became the largest cocaine producer in the world. During the 1990s, it also became the largest coca grower nation. Furthermore, Colombia produces and supplies the lion's share of heroin consumed in the United States and also exports illegal marijuana.

Illegal drug production and trafficking in Colombia have marked the past thirty years of the country's history. In no other country has the illegal drug industry had such dramatic social, political, and economic effects. Illegal drugs have contributed greatly to changes in institutions and values, have indirectly conditioned the country's economic performance, and have become a major element in the country's policy. Illegal drug revenues are a primary source of funds for left- and right-wing armed actors of the ambiguous war currently experienced in the country.

This article summarizes the development of the illegal drug industry and attempts to identify its main effects on Colombia and the government's main reactions and policies in response to it.

ILLEGAL DRUG INDUSTRY DEVELOPMENT

Marijuana

Illegal drug production and trafficking started to grow in Colombia in the mid-1960s when marijuana crops developed in response to increases in domestic demand, which echoed American developments. Still, marijuana production and traffic did not become important until the early 1970s. The growth in marijuana consumption in the United States and Europe in the 1960s triggered the development of large marijuana plantings in Mexico and Jamaica to supply them. Toward the end of the decade, the U.S. government promoted eradication programs in Mexico using paraquat, a herbicide known to have harmful health effects, which drew away American consumers. This measure created strong incentives to find other marijuana-growing sites, and the marijuana crop was then displaced to Colombia.

Marijuana grew mainly in the Sierra Nevada de Santa Marta on Colombia's Caribbean coast. At the beginning, American smugglers sought Colombian suppliers. Some local and American entrepreneurs provided seeds to poor peasants from whom they obtained the marijuana to be sold to the Americans. After a short time, "Colombians seized the opportunity offered by the new market, and rapidly replaced the Americans organizing production to become marijuana exporters, but Americans retained marketing control" (Thoumi 1995, 126). News about the good marijuana business spread rapidly, and by the late 1970s, marijuana plantings had appeared in several other regions, particularly in isolated, recently settled areas of the country (Ruiz-Hernández 1979).

Marijuana-exporting organizations were relatively simple. The peasants produced for a local exporter who controlled and/or owned one or a few landing strips or a port and negotiated with the American importer. Due to the lack of land titling and the very rudimentary and uncompetitive capital markets, the exporter frequently provided crop financing (Ruiz-Hernández 1979, 140). Most peasants in the Sierra Nevada de Santa Marta had roots in that area, and many of them retired from the illegal business after a couple of successful crops provided them with enough capital to maintain a satisfactory living standard growing legal crops (Ruiz-Hernández 1979, 140).

The illegal marijuana boom, victim to several external forces, started to decline in 1978. In late 1978, the U.S. government questioned President Turbay's antidrug credentials because of possible links between traffickers and some of his close political supporters. In response, the Colombian government engaged in an aggressive manual eradication campaign, confiscated boats and airplanes, and destroyed some of the marijuana processing equipment (Thoumi 1995, chap. 3). By that time, marijuana production in the United States had grown substantially after

the development of the more potent *sin semilla* variety.

These developments made the marijuana business less attractive, but they did not destroy it. Moreover, marijuana had infused Colombian entrepreneurs with the awareness of other potential illegal sources of wealth. Methaqualone began to be produced or imported and then exported jointly with marijuana (Ruiz-Hernández 1979, 180).

Marijuana did not disappear, but as the cocaine industry developed, the policy focus shifted away from it. This changed in May 1984 after Minister of Justice Rodrigo Lara-Bonilla was assassinated and President Betancur used aerial spraying against marijuana plantings. Traffickers' response to fumigation was to shift the location of marijuana plantings to locations characterized by lack of state presence and a very high level of violence. In several of these regions, guerrilla organizations rooted out the bullies, established order, and gained peasants' support (Vargas 1994). Marijuana eradication campaigns continued during the 1980s with American support, and by 1990, marijuana plantings were relatively marginal in Colombia (U.S. Department of State 1992, 104). Uribe (1997) concluded that in the mid-1990s, there were about six thousand hectares planted with marijuana concentrated in six regions of the country used to satisfy mostly the domestic demand.

Coca and cocaine

Cocaine is a more appealing trafficking drug than marijuana because it has much higher value to weight and volume ratios and because coca cannot be produced in Europe or the United States, except in a few areas in Puerto Rico, Hawaii, and Guam. To grow coca does not require special skills; the plant is very hardy and fits very well in fragile tropical soils, and cocaine manufacturing is a simple process.

In the mid-1970s, illegal entrepreneurs began to export small quantities of cocaine to the United States. Very high profits quickly allowed the business to become self-financing and to expand and induced Colombians to develop (1) stable routes and links with coca paste suppliers from Bolivia and Peru and with suppliers of chemical inputs to refine cocaine and (2) transportation systems to make large shipments and distribution networks, especially in the United States. The large number of Colombian immigrants facilitated this. The growth of the illegal business promoted the development of increasingly sophisticated money-laundering systems enabled in part by the large and complex contraband networks used to import many goods into Colombia.

The illegal traffic was a strong incentive for the development of coca plantings in Colombia, which appeared as a backward linkage of the cocaine trade during the mid-1970s (Thoumi 1995, chap. 3). By 1987, Colombia produced 11 percent of the world's coca crop (Sarmiento 1990, 69-70). Coca's production has had an upward, albeit unstable, long-term trend. Coca prices have fallen in the long run and at times, when the government has intensified its

antidrug fight against the cartels, they have collapsed, generating deep depressions in coca-growing regions because of the disruption of coca leaf demand.

During the twentieth century, Colombia suffered several internal conflict episodes that forced significant domestic peasant displacements. Coca plantings in Colombia developed almost exclusively in areas recently settled by displaced peasants where the state has a weak, if any, presence. These regions are isolated and distant from the main economic centers of the country.

During the 1990s, the number of coca plantings exploded in Colombia. In 1991, Colombia was the third largest coca-growing nation with 18.8 percent of the Andean countries' coca acreage but produced only 13.7 percent of the coca leaf volume (Thoumi 1995, chap. 3). In 1995, there were 80,000 hectares of coca in Colombia (Uribe 1997), more than double the 1990 figure. The increase continued during the late 1990s, reaching some 120,000 to 150,000 hectares by 2000. This, coupled with substantial declines in the area cultivated in Peru and Bolivia, turned Colombia into the largest coca-producing country in the world. Furthermore, cocaine yields increased significantly as growers and refiners adopted important technological advances (Uribe 1997).

Several factors should be mentioned as contributors to the 1990s coca boom. First, the Fujimori administration, with American support, developed an illegal flight interdiction program that dried up coca paste supply to Colombia. Second, the collapse of the iron curtain weakened the finances of Fuerzas Armadas Revolucionarios de Columbia (FARC) (Revolutionary Armed Forces of Colombia) guerrillas who sought alternative funding in the illegal industry. Third, paramilitary and guerrillas found it useful to promote illegal plantings to develop and keep peasant support in the areas they controlled.

The coca boom incorporated a complex set of new actors to the illegal industry. In coca-growing areas, guerrilla and paramilitary groups substitute for the state in imposing a very authoritarian regime, defining and applying their own laws and regulations, and providing education, police, and civil justice to solve conflicts among the population. In exchange, these groups charge coca production and cocaine export taxes (Uribe 1997; Vargas 1999). Other actors include longtime settlers who moved to the region to follow their farmer vocations, produce mainly foodstuffs, and devote a small part of their land to coca and recent settlers who devote most of their efforts to producing coca paste but also devote some of their land to coca. Finally, there are recent migrants who arrive in the region to grow coca (González-Arias 1998, 52-53). There are also commercial farmers with large plantings between twenty-five and two hundred hectares who have direct links with traffickers; many of them own laboratories. Most workers in these farms are *raspachines* who pick coca leaves and help in the manufacturing process. González-Arias (1998) argued that this is a heterogeneous group made up of displaced peasants, former rural hired workers and pickers who came from regions that produce coffee or modern agriculture crops and who expect to settle in coca-growing regions, and transient raspachines who expect to make some money before returning to their places of origin.

Until recently, coca was processed into paste by peasants themselves and *chichipatos* who gather paste to sell in small quantities to *traquetos*. These furnished the links to trafficking organizations (González-Arias 1998, 53). There is also a group of parachuters who do not live in the region and fly small planes to come in and out. They bring large amounts of cash (pesos or dollars) and buy big quantities of cocaine from the large "factories" and traquetos.

In late 1998, the Pastrana administration granted the FARC guerrillas control over a large part of the country where coca plantings were widespread. To a large extent, the guerrillas have substituted the chichipatos and traquetos and have profited from selling to trafficking organizations. A similar situation has developed in paramilitary-controlled coca regions. While illegal drugs are a main source of funds for these groups, involvement in international drug trafficking is impossible to determine at the time.

The illegal industry has also generated a strong illicit chemical input and arms trade. These products are extremely hard to control. Besides, once the industry establishes export-smuggling capabilities, it also can import many products using many of the same smuggling systems.[1]

Poppy, opium, and heroin

Poppy cultivation was first detected in Colombia in 1986. Available evidence indicates that traffickers who distributed seeds and guaranteed crop purchases to traditional peasants in minifundia high-altitude regions promoted poppy plantings. Many of these peasants belong to Indian communities. Poppy plantings spread quickly over many areas of the Colombian Andes (Vargas and Barragán 1995). In traditional Indian areas, poppy has increased peasants' incomes but has created conflicts over payments, created misunderstandings about business transactions, and attracted undesirable outsiders to the growing areas where violence has increased (Vargas and Barragán 1995). These developments have disrupted communities and have challenged their ancestral authority structures. In these communities, many prominent elders support eradication negotiations.

Poppy has also attracted non-Indian migrants to high-altitude unsettled regions and has been a main cause of high-altitude old primary forest destruction. Guerrilla presence has also increased in poppy-growing regions. Poppy grows in "commercial" and "peasant" plantings (Uribe 1997). The commercial ones are generally in vacant government lands, and growers use modern techniques, fertilizers, herbicides, and fungicides, many of which are sold by drug buyers. These generally do not exceed a total of five hectares divided in several small plots to avoid detection. Commercial plantings employ hired labor while peasant plantings employ only family labor, use less sophisticated production techniques, and are less profitable.

Traffickers do not buy opium in Colombia because they cannot guarantee purity. Instead, morphine base is refined near poppy plantings where it is sold to traffickers (Uribe 1997). Estimates of poppy, morphine, and heroin production are very weak partly because poppy is a short-cycle crop. Several estimates (Uribe 1997; Vargas 1999) show poppy plantings between six thousand and twenty thousand hectares during the 1990s. In any case, these are sufficient to supply a significant share of the U.S. heroin demand.

Cartels, marketing networks, guerrillas, and paramilitary

Criminal networks are in constant flux to avoid detection. They continuously seek new routes, sources of chemical inputs, ways to disguise exports, and channels to influence politicians. High profits and low barriers to entry continuously attract independent operators that spring up at various stages of the business.

Marijuana development did not result in complex business enterprises. These came to life with cocaine, which started as a small-scale artisan activity but quickly became a sophisticated business activity. This was the result of a more elaborate production process, the need to import unrefined cocaine from other countries, and the greater profit incentives. The development of large-scale smuggling methods increased potential gains dramatically and induced the formation of cartels or export syndicates.

These export syndicates were organized to spread risk and guarantee profits. They coordinated the Colombian cocaine industry. They sent coca paste and cocaine base buyers to Bolivia and Peru where they organized shipments to Colombia, established laboratories to refine cocaine or subcontracted that process, and organized the illegal exports from Colombia and the wholesale of the product in the United States and other markets. The extremely high profits of the cocaine business induced Colombians to participate in all stages of the cocaine industry, including its distribution in the United States where the large number of Colombian immigrants facilitated the establishment of distribution networks. This development was also facilitated by the proclivity of Colombians to use violence against other smuggling organizations. Violence was also instrumental in deterring the development of export syndicates in Bolivia and Peru from competing with Colombians.

The large profits generated by the illegal industry also required the development of sophisticated money-laundering systems. Rapid wealth acquisition, furthermore, made it impossible for successful exporters not to be noticed. Their high notoriety increased their need for a social support network to protect their business, illegal profits, and accumulated capital. One of the early strategies for social support was to let wealthy Colombians buy shares in a cocaine shipment, under a system known as *la apuntada* (Krauthausen and Sarmiento 1991, 74).

The illegal drug industry comprised peasants, chemists, various types of suppliers, purchasers and intermediaries, pilots, lawyers, financial and tax advisers, enforcers, bodyguards, front men (*testaferros*), and smugglers who help launder profits. They were tied to the central cartels in different ways. Some were directly part of the cartels, but many were independent subcontractors loosely tied to them. The network also included politicians, police, guerrillas, paramilitaries, individual army members, public employees, bankers, loyal relatives, friends, childhood friends, and others. The social support network provides protection to the illegal industry, mostly at a price, and constitutes the main channel through which the illegal industry penetrated and corrupted social institutions. Through this network, illegal income was distributed to the rest of society and forged strong loyalties within the illegal industry.

During the 1980s, the Medellín and Cali cartels gained notoriety in international cocaine markets. In reality, these were not truly cartels with the capacity to exclude and control production but rather were syndicates that improved the efficiency of distribution. Smaller syndicates remained in the shadow of the two main ones. These varied from relatively large organizations to mom-and-pop organizations that exported small quantities. Most information about export organizations focuses on the Medellín and Cali cartels, and little is known about the rest.

During the 1990s, the Colombian illegal drug industry experienced significant structural alterations in response to changes in demand or government policies. First, cocaine demand in the United States stagnated while cocaine production increased. The resulting lower prices encouraged traffickers to search for new markets and products.[2] Trafficking organizations became more international, and links were established between Colombian and European criminal organizations (Clawson and Lee 1996, 62-90). Second, increased U.S. interdiction efforts in the Caribbean led to a routing shift to Mexico and the development of links between Colombian and Mexican traffickers. The latter increased their market share at the expense of the former. Third, after the 1989 assassination of the leading presidential candidate Luis Carlos Galán, the Barco and Gaviria governments followed a war against narcoterrorism that destroyed the Medellín cartel. Pressured by the United States, the following Samper government fought the Cali cartel and incarcerated all its leaders. Fourth, as the two large cartels were weakened, a large number of smaller trafficking organizations sprouted up. These have followed low-profile strategies, are led by more educated Colombians, and are more difficult to track down. Fifth, these smaller organizations are also functional for heroin smuggling. Heroin has a substantially higher price per kilo than cocaine, and its volume demand in the United States is much smaller. These two factors make heroin an ideal trafficking drug for small

criminal organizations. Seventh, coca and poppy planting boomed. This added new actors and complexity to the drug industry, particularly paramilitary and guerrilla organizations that use illegal drugs as a main funding source.

THE SIZE OF THE ILLEGAL INDUSTRY AND ITS ECONOMIC EFFECTS ON THE COUNTRY

Size is one of the determinants of an illegal activity's effects on a country. The illegality of the industry makes estimating its size quite difficult. Every estimate requires many assumptions about key variables such as cocaine content in coca leaves, chemists' skills, smuggling costs, and so on. Not surprisingly, available estimates show a wide variation depending on the particular assumptions made.[3] The most rigorous estimates place total illegal drug value added in the $2 billion to $4 billion range in the early and mid-1980s and somewhat less afterward. During the 1990s, these estimates placed total illegal drug value added at around $2.5 billion per year, but they did not include possible profits repatriated by Colombian traffickers abroad.

In the early and mid-1980s, GNP was about $36 billion, measured in current dollars. During the 1990s, it grew substantially to $68.6 billion in 1994 and $96.3 billion in 1997.[4] According to these estimates, the value added generated by the illegal drug industry in the early 1980s was in the 7 to 10 percent GNP range, but by the late 1990s, it dropped to 3 to 4 percent. These estimates show that the relative importance of the illegal industry in the Colombian economy has been declining. One important issue is the question, What has been the effect of the illegal industry on the Colombian economy?

There is no doubt that the impact of the industry on Colombia has been quite large. The private-sector capital formation during the 1980s averaged $2.8 billion a year (Thoumi 1995). Furthermore, any criminal organization exporting fifty or more tons of cocaine a year would have profits that compete with those of the largest financial conglomerates of the country.[5] Any estimate of the size and profits of the illegal drug industry, no matter how conservative, highlights the capacity of the illegal drug industry to change the economic power structure of the country (Thoumi 1995).

The effects of illegal revenues and profits on the Colombian economy have evolved through time. During the 1970s and 1980s, they generated real estate booms in a few cities and regions, revalued the Colombian peso, and encouraged contraband imports. The illegal export boom was welcomed by most Colombians who for decades had confronted a tight foreign exchange constraint.

It can be argued that the drug industry has penetrated many economic activities, particularly rural and urban real estate; however, a very large part of the Colombian economy, including its most modern enterprises, have been rather insulated from the illegal industry power. The modern Colombian economy has been controlled by a number of financial conglomerates that include financial, manufacturing, modern agricultural, marketing, and media organizations. These groups tend to be self-contained and have a lot to lose developing partnerships with illicit entrepreneurs. Furthermore, the stock market is very thin, and most companies traded are controlled by those financial conglomerates. Not surprisingly, there are few activities in which large sums of illicit funds can be laundered in Colombia. Indeed, the "laundromat is quite small" (Thoumi 1999).

While the illegal drug industry has been important, it cannot be argued that the performance of the Colombian economy has improved because of the drug income. Indeed, the Colombian GNP's rate of growth during the postcocaine era (1980 on) through 1997 was about 3.2 percent, while it averaged 5.5 percent during the thirty years before. This decline cannot be explained by the Latin American foreign debt crisis of the 1980s, which Colombia avoided, or by worse international terms of trade or other external conditions during the 1980s than during the three earlier decades (Thoumi 1995). After 1995, the performance of the Colombian economy declined sharply, and in 1999, it registered a decline of about 5 percent of GDP. This was the first year since the end of World War II in which income fell.

When the illegal industry began to grow, its short-run effects on the economy tended to be positive but in the medium and long run, its effects have been highly negative. The drug industry has acted as a catalyst that accelerated a process of "delegit-imation of the regime" that has contributed to the country's stagnation (Thoumi 1995). This process produced a sharp decline in trust that increased transaction costs, contributed to increased violence and impunity that has induced "clean" capital flight and larger security costs, promoted expectations of very fast wealth accumulation that produced highly speculative investments and increases in bankruptcies, embezzlements, and so forth. Increased criminality has had a significant declining effect on the country's income growth rate: "The cost of crime in terms of lost growth exceeded 2 percent per year, without including its longer term effects on factor productivity and capital formation" (Rubio 1996, 32).

During the 1990s, the negative effects became sharply noticeable when illegal drugs became a main funding source for right- and left-wing guerrilla and right-wing paramilitary movements. Today, a significant part of illicit revenues is used to buy weapons and pay warriors. It is ironic that when the illegal drug revenues are received by guerrilla and paramilitary groups and fund the ambiguous war in progress and when they are received by government and military officers, they go to private pockets. In all cases, they greatly undermine the state and the licit economy. The illicit industry thus became a main immediate cause of the current Colombian social crises and also contributes to the destruction of productive activities and to capital flight.

THE ILLEGAL INDUSTRY'S EFFECTS ON POLITICS

The political system has been more vulnerable than the country's economy to the power of the illegal industry. The illegal industry has had to develop social and political support networks to protect its investments and to prevent the government from jailing traffickers and, more important, extraditing them to the United States. They have used carrot-and-stick strategies to obtain these means.

Extradition has been the main source of conflict between the government and drug traffickers who have used all available resources to fight it. This was the main cause of the narco-terrorism that erupted in the late 1980s and that included the assassination of many prominent politicians including several presidential candidates.

In the early 1980s, members of the Medellín cartel tried to obtain power directly and developed a strong support base, spending some of their wealth in public works. Pablo Escobar "bought" a politician and got himself elected to the Colombian Congress as a backup.[6] Carlos Lehder established a small nationalist party that did not prosper. The Medellín cartel invested heavily in rural land and promoted the formation of self-protection paramilitary. The Medellín cartel did not hesitate to use violence against the public who opposed it or who simply tried to enforce laws as their duties required. The need to influence government policies also induced traffickers to develop links with politicians. Their wealth allowed them to make large political contributions. Not surprisingly, jointly with the large financial conglomerates, they became the main contributors to political campaigns.

By the late 1970s, the illegal industry was already a large election-funding source, and the industry contributed heavily to the 1982 election.[7] The 1986 and 1990 presidential and congressional campaigns were fairly free of illicit drug funding because at the time the government was waging the war against narcoterrorism. In 1994, the large amounts of illegal industry funds received by the Samper campaign became a main political and international issue that crippled the government and produced an unprecedented political crisis.

The benefits that drug traffickers have obtained from their contributions to politicians are debatable. On one hand, many drug traffickers, including the leaders of the old Medellín and Cali syndicates were jailed or killed. Besides, despite large campaign funding, President Samper was forced by American pressures to implement very strong repressive policies against the illegal industry. This led Gutiérrez-Sanín (2001) to argue that traffickers did not get much for their money. On the other hand, most traffickers avoided extradition, and many have continued to run their business from jail. A few points are worth mentioning in regard to this issue. While drug moneys can cover a very large share of a political campaign, they are insignificant relative to total drug revenues. This means that traffickers are willing to throw away funds to politicians without a quid pro quo determined at the time of the contributions. As noted by Lee and Thoumi (1999), many traffickers simply use their contributions as a "joker" that they can pull out when needed later on. Besides, many inconspicuous nonextraditable traffickers use their contributions just to gain social recognition.

COLOMBIAN POLICIES AND ATTITUDES

Colombia is in the midst of an institutional crisis characterized by extremely low levels of social capital and trust. It is a country where society imposes very few behavioral constraints on its members. Indeed, every Colombian has to develop his or her own ethical norms. Not surprisingly, Colombia is a country of "individual creativity and social indiscipline" (Gómez-Buendía 1999, 20). This environment produces extreme individual behaviors and exceptional individuals, some of whom go to any extreme to comply with the law and others to break it. Success in Colombia is individual but not collective. Loyalty is extended to those close to oneself because it is necessary to survive in a hostile institutional environment. "The net result is the abundance of antisocial conducts and the preponderance of private over collective rationality" (p. 20).

Not surprisingly, during the past fifty years, Colombia was the country of muddle-through policies. Policy changes were gradual and motivated by the individual interests of those in power. Social reforms deemed necessary by many intellectuals and foreign observers were at best enacted but weakly implemented so that they did not achieve their social goals. These were the cases of rural land tenancy, education, and tax reforms.

The weak government confronted many policy issues: very rapid urbanization; great pressures to provide education, housing, and health services to its population; and great pressures to promote food production, create infrastructure, and so forth. Individual addiction to psychoactive drugs was (and is) a very low priority issue on the government's agenda. Besides, individual addiction is perceived mainly as a personal problem. Most Colombians did not realistically expect to have the government take care of it. Indeed, "as long as it does not concern me directly, it is not my problem."[8]

In Colombia,

impersonal norms exist and are recognized except that they are not taken seriously, there is a low law breaking threshold, and many consider "my case an exceptional one" that requires me to break or dodge the law. This constitutes a sort of democracy in which we are all equal because we have the right to evade or avoid the law. (Gómez-Buendía 1999, 20)

In this case, if drugs are a foreign problem, why should Colombians take care of it?

Policies followed by the Colombian government at various times cover the full spectrum of repressive measures used against drug trafficking. These include the jailing and extraditing of traffickers; involuntary eradication of illicit crops and alternative development programs for affected peasants; import, production, and marketing controls of chemical inputs used to refine cocaine and heroin; interdiction of illicit drugs; anti-money-laundering measures in the financial system; and seizure and confiscation of assets. On the demand side, there are also addiction treatment policies.

The implementation of these policies has been affected by government priorities and weaknesses and the structural limitations of the policies themselves. Consider first eradication. Colombia is the only country where aerial spraying takes place. This is done because the government does not have a strong presence or control over the regions in question. This policy generates a strong opposition from environmentalists and peasants and has not succeeded in limiting illegal crop acreage; rather, it has contributed to planting displacement around the country.

Alternative development programs have been attempted in Colombia. Unfortunately, it is difficult to think of a country where these are less likely to succeed. Coca plantings are in areas with very poor and fragile soils, inaccessible by highway, and far away from any realistic market. Peasants are relatively recent settlers, have weak community institutions, and are armed. All this makes it difficult to negotiate any program and to find real alternative crops. Indeed, whether there should be any agricultural activity in those areas is a big question.

Traffickers are imprisoned, but the state has very little control over what goes on inside jails and prisons. They are overcrowded and underfunded, prisoners have access to cellular phones, and weekly visitors smuggle arms, weapons, and other items. Prisons are understaffed, and personnel are poorly paid. Inmates organize themselves in gangs and many actually build facilities within the jail. Escapes are common, and many traffickers have been able to continue running their business while in prison.

Expropriations of traffickers' assets had been seen as a key policy against organized crime and a source of funds for antidrug policies. The government simply does not have the financial and managerial capacity to administer seized property, and expropriation procedures are complex, costly, and difficult to implement successfully. The Colombian drug control office (Dirección Nacional de Estupefacientes) in charge of handling these properties is woefully inadequate to do the job. Only a handful of properties have been expropriated, and lawyers have had a field day defending traffickers and their heirs against the state.[9]

When the illegal drug industry started, it was very difficult to mobilize public opinion against something that was not perceived as a social threat. The first eradication campaigns in the late 1970s were pursued in response to American pressures on the government. An extradition treaty was signed with the United States in the late seventies and ratified in 1982, but the government did not enforce it until the assassination of a minister of justice by the drug traffickers. In other

words, antidrug policies for many years were reactive either to foreign pressures or misdeeds by the illegal industry. The wave of terror that followed generated a strong anti-extradition sentiment among the population so that extradition was declared unconstitutional in the new 1991 constitution.[10]

Until the late 1980s, most Colombians did not perceive the negative long-term effects of the illegal industry, and public support for antidrug policies was weak. During the 1980s, homicides and other violent crimes increased dramatically, and by 1989, it was evident to most Colombians that the illegal industry's effects on the political system were perverse. During the 1990s, it became clear that the illegal industry was funding both guerrillas and paramilitary groups. Contrary to what has happened in some Central American countries and Vietnam, guerrilla groups do not have strong social support. Colombian guerrillas in many ways represent Colombia's past, not its future. They are rural based in a country 75 percent urban, their level of education is very low in a country where literacy rates increased sharply, and they use violence and primitive conflict resolution methods in a society that aspires to modern social institutions. Furthermore, Colombia is subject to strong external pressures, and Colombians are discriminated against around the world (Colombian profiling is legal and legitimate all over the world). Today, Colombians realize that the illegal industry was a catalyst in a process of social decomposition, but since their institutions are so weak, there is little they individually can do about it.

Notes

1. Many inputs are bulkier, which is a disincentive to use small planes to smuggle them. However, traffickers smuggle inputs selectively depending on which are harder to find in Colombian markets.

2. Steiner (1997, 35) used Drug Enforcement Administration data and estimated the midrange wholesale price per kilogram in the United States at $60,000 in 1980, $40,000 in 1985, $25,500 in 1990, and $22,500 in 1990. Prices in Miami had been significantly lower.

3. These have been surveyed by Thoumi (1995) and Steiner (1997), among others.

4. These figures are based on the Inter-American Development Bank online database.

5. A back-of-the-envelope estimate can place export profits net of transportation costs at about $10,000 per kilogram or $500 million per 50 tons. SEMANA (Los cuatro grandes 1996) estimated that in 1995, the four largest financial groups had profits of $530 million, $140 million, $480 million, and $190 million. After 1998, Colombia entered a deep recession, and the profits of these conglomerates have suffered drastically.

6. At the time, every congressperson had a backup who would replace the elected candidate when he or she was absent.

7. Lee and Thoumi (1999) studied this issue in detail. Former president Alfonso López-Michelsen (2001) acknowledged in a newly published book that his 1982 campaign received about $400,000 from the illegal industry. This is a remarkable confession because the total campaign cost that year did not likely exceed $1 million.

8. It should be noted that despite a very low street price of about $5 a gram, cocaine use in Colombia is not perceived as an epidemic. The most detailed survey (Pérez 2000) found that in 1999-2000, 1.4 percent of the youth between fifteen and nineteen had used cocaine in the past month and 4.4 percent had used it at least once in their lives. These figures are not particularly low, but they do not generate a social reaction comparable to that of the United States.

9. *El Tiempo*, the country's main newspaper, reported on 9 May 2001 that only thirty-three of thirty-four thousand seized properties had been expropriated. The government does not have an inventory of seized assets, many looted and burned properties would cost very large sums to fix, and others continue to be exploited by their owners who now do not pay taxes or maintain them. In some cases, armed paramilitary groups prevent the government from taking possession of seized assets. The potential cost to the government arising from litigation can be enormous.

10. A constitutional amendment has since changed this.

References

Clawson, Patrick L., and Rensselaer Lee III. 1996. *The Andean cocaine industry*. New York: St. Martin's.

Gómez-Buendía, Hernando. 1999. La Hipótesis del Almendrón. In *¿Para Dónde Va Colombia?*, edited by Hernando Gómez-Buendía. Bogota, Colombia: TM Editores-Colciencias.

González-Arias, José J. 1998. Cultivos ilícitos, colonización y revuelta de raspachines. *Revista Foro* 35 (September).

Gutiérrez-Sanín, Francisco. 2001. Organized crime and the political system in Colombia (1978-1998). Paper presented at the Conference on Democracy, Human Rights and Peace in Colombia, Kellogg Institute, University of Notre Dame, Indiana, 26-27 March.

Krauthausen, Ciro, and Luis F. Sarmiento. 1991. *Cocaína & Co.: Un mercado ilegal por dentro*. Bogota, Colombia: Tercer Mundo Editores.

Lee, Rensselaer W. III, and Francisco E. Thoumi. 1999. The criminal-political nexus in Colombia. *Trends in Organized Crime* 5 (2).

López-Michelsen, Alfonso. 2001. *Palabras pendientes (conversaciones con Enrique Santos-Calderón)*. Bogota, Colombia: El Ancora Editores.

Los cuatro grandes. 1996. *SEMANA* 731:56-64.

Pérez, Augusto. 2000. *Sondeo nacional del consumo de dorgas en jóvenes, 1999-2000.* Bogota, Colombia: Programa Presidencial Rumbos.

Rubio, Mauricio. 1996. Crimen y crecimiento en Colombia. In *Hacia un enfoque integrado del desarrollo: Ética, violencia y seguridad ciudadana, encuentro de reflexión.* Washington, DC: Inter-American Development Bank.

Ruiz-Hernández, Hernando. 1979. Implicaciones sociales y económicas de la producción de la marihuana. In *Marihuana: Legalización o represión,* edited by Asociación Nacional de Instituciones Financieras. Bogota, Colombia: Biblioteca ANIF de Economía.

Sarmiento, Eduardo. 1990. Economía del Narcotráfico. In *Narcotráfico en Colombia: Dimensiones políticas, económicas, jurídicas e internacionales,* edited by C. G. Arrieta et al. Tercer Mundo Editores-Ediciones Uniandes.

Steiner, Roberto. 1997. *Los dólares del narcotráfico.* Cuadernos de fedesarrollo no. 2. Bogota, Colombia: Tercer Mundo Editores.

Thoumi, Francisco E. 1995. *Political economy and illegal drugs in Colombia.* Boulder, CO: Lynne Rienner.

————. 1999. La relación entre corrupción y narcotráfico: Un análisis general y algunas referencias a Colombia. *Revista de Economía del Rosario* 2 (1).

Uribe, Sergio. 1997. Los cultivos ilícitos en Colombia. Evaluación: Extensión, técnicas y tecnologías para la producción y rendimientos y magnitud de la industria. In *Drogas ilícitas en Colombia: Su impacto económico, político y social,* edited by F. Thoumi. Bogota, Colombia: Editorial Planeta.

U.S. Department of State, Bureau of International Narcotics Matters. 1992. *International narcotics control strategy report.* Washington, DC: Department of State Publication 9948-A.

Vargas, Ricardo. 1994. La bonanza de la marimba empezó aquí. In *La verdad del '93: Paz, derechos humanos y violencia.* Bogota, Colombia: CINEP.

————. 1999. *Drogas máscaras y juegos. Narcotráfico y conflicto armado en Colombia.* Bogota, Colombia: TM Editores- TNI-Acción Andina.

Vargas, Ricardo, and Jacqueline Barragán. 1995. Amapola en Colombia: Economía ilegal, violencias e impacto regional. In *Drogas poder y región en Colombia,* vol. 2, edited by R. Vargas. Bogota, Colombia: CINEP.

Policy Paradox:
Implications of U.S. Drug
Control Policy for Jamaica

By MARLYN J. JONES

ABSTRACT: U.S. drug control policies impose supply reduction targets on source and transit nations without regard for their social, economic, or political environments. Simultaneously, immigration policies deport drug felons to these countries. This article advances the argument that these policies have displaced responsibility for U.S. crime problems. As a result, there is displacement of criminal activities to areas of least resistance, with drug transit nations being disproportionately affected. The article addresses, in part, the paucity of drug policy literature on the Caribbean drug transit region. It discusses the nexus between U.S. drug and immigration policies and the resulting consequences for Jamaica, a drug transit country. Jamaica is of special interest because of its long-standing presence on the U.S. drug policy agenda and its stereotyping in journalistic discussions.

Marlyn J. Jones is a criminologist at California State University, Sacramento, where she serves as assistant professor in the Division of Criminal Justice. Her research interests include Caribbean criminology, policy analysis, and issues of race and gender.

THE perception that ethnics and foreigners are primarily responsible for America's drug problems creates a nexus between drug and immigration policies. This nexus materializes as a dominant policy issue between the United States and its western hemispheric neighbors. This happens because the U.S. government considers illicit drugs and illegal immigration terrorist enterprises that undermine its national security.

Deportation has emerged as the panacea for drug and crime problems. Consequently, individuals, many of whom were convicted on drug-related offences, are being deported to drug-producing and/or transit nations that must be constantly cognizant of U.S.-imposed drug policy targets. The issue for U.S. policy consideration is how to manage tradeoffs between these goals. Instead of asking why the United States should keep deportable felons, I suggest that this question should be revised. Rather, one should ask whether the United States is achieving its articulated goals. And even if the goals are being achieved, are the consequences of the policy unjustifiable? Herein I argue that the supply reduction goals are not being achieved and the underlying premises of the supply reduction policy are unrealistic and unrealizable. A primary result is the displacement of drug-related crime and violence into, and the exacerbation of economic problems in, areas of least resistance.

U.S. DRUG POLICY

A basic objective of U.S. counternarcotics policy is to bolster political will in the key source and transit countries. The intent is to prevent drug interests from becoming entrenched. As stated in the 2000 *International Narcotics Control Strategy Report* (INCSR) (http://www.state.gov/g/inl/rls/nrcrpt/2000/index.cfm?docid=886),

In those nations where political leaders have had the courage to sacrifice short-term economic and political considerations in favor of the long-term national interest, we have seen the drug trade falter. And where political will has wavered, we have seen the drug syndicates flourish and corruption set in.

Consequently, supply reduction at the source has become the cornerstone of a U.S. drug policy that also advocates the creation of a drug-free America by 2007. This mandate was reenforced by the United Nations General Assembly Special Session on Drugs in its 1998 declaration for a drug-free world by 2008.

Two of the four primary assumptions of the drug policy about supply reduction at the source are the following:

1. Production and distribution of illicit-drugs in the source zone can be controlled and reduced by appropriate crop control, economic development, legal and institutional reforms, international cooperation, and demand reduction activities.

2. Political, economic and social instability in the countries of the source and transit zones will not prevent host governments from pursuing effective drug control efforts. (Performance Management Evaluation 2000, Appendix E-109)

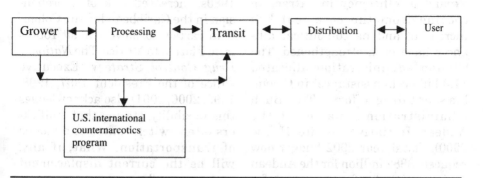

FIGURE 1
FIVE-POINT GROWER-TO-USER CONTINUUM

The INCSR also states that supply reduction initiatives focus on critical points along a five-point grower-to-user chain linking the consumer in the United States to the grower in a source country (see Figure 1).

A primary supply reduction goal is to prevent drugs from entering the United States. While this is a noble and worthwhile gesture, because the international counternarcotics program emphasizes the first three links, success in curtailing the entry of drugs into the United States will have a disproportionate effect at the terminating or transit point. Yet despite a plethora of drug policy literature focusing on source countries, little if any information currently exists on drug policy consequences at transit points. It becomes important therefore to assess the feasibility of U.S. drug policy assumptions and evaluate the imposition of antidrug targets at transit zones.

Failure to achieve U.S. drug control targets has a range of consequences, such as decertification. Certification is the U.S. government's annual assessment of whether governments of major drug-producing countries and transit zones have cooperated fully with the United States. The certification process also assesses whether countries have taken adequate steps on their own to meet the goals and objectives of the 1988 United Nations drug convention. Noncomplying countries may be decertified. Decertification involves the withdrawal of all but humanitarian and antinarcotic aid and the withholding of U.S. vote from international funding agencies such as the International Monetary Fund. Decertification has economic consequences; however, supply reduction targets are implemented without regard for the social, political, and economic environment in which these societies operate. The supply reduction assumptions also incorporate the supposition that the United Nations will not change the schedule for drugs. Cumulatively, the impositions and suppositions lead one to question whether they impose undue hardship on the targeted countries.

The 2000 INCSR states that in Colombia, which produces the bulk of illicit narcotics entering the United States, coca cultivation has expanded, efficiency in extracting cocaine from the coca leaf has increased, and narco-political alliances have been strengthened. The Clinton administration allocated $1.3 billion in assistance[1] to Colombia's antidrug efforts. The Bush administration renamed it the Andean Initiative (White House 2000). Fiscal year 2002 budget now requests $882 million for the Andean region, with half earmarked for Colombia (Bureau of Western Hemispheric Fact Sheet 2001). Will these initiatives in Colombia lead to displacement and thereby exacerbate problems in neighboring countries?

DISPLACEMENT

Displacement refers to an empirical phenomenon that implies that efforts to suppress criminality result in compensating behavior. Accordingly, changes occur when there is increased law enforcement directed at one area. Gabor (1981) suggested that crime displacement, or adjustments to circumvent preventive measures, can occur along three dimensions—spatial, temporal, or qualitative. These involve a mass shift in criminal activity from one type of crime to another or from one geographical area to another.

The drug control arena exhibits a high degree of displacement, such as shifts in the method of operation, changes in geographical areas of operation, or criminal movement away from drug-related activities. Flexibility in trafficking and distribution routes contributes to geographical displacement. Smith (1992, 13) noted that during the 1980s, increased risk of apprehension in the Caribbean led the Colombian cartels to move transit routes from Florida to Mexico. The *National Drug Control Strategy* (Executive Office of the President 1997, 1998, 1999, 2000, 2001) also acknowledges this flexibility, stating that traffickers often switch routes and modes of transportation. What, if any, will be the current displacement consequences?

Arganaras (1997) identified three main harmful effects of previous U.S. counternarcotics policy in Bolivia, a source country. These included the institutionalization of a permanent army of unwaged laborers, the militarization of law enforcement, and the devaluation of political goods in the formal democracy. Craig (1987), in an assessment of drug-producing states, also found social, economic, and political consequences of illicit narcotics control for the source countries. These include violence within the country, corruption at all levels, and economic effects that had penetrated many aspects of the society. Political consequences were most evident in the government's inability to control outlying areas and loss of legitimacy for failure to control such trafficking or to enforce the rule of law within the country (Craig 1987, 2).

JAMAICA AS A U.S. FOREIGN (DRUG) POLICY CONCERN

Early drug policy literature identified Jamaica as one of three primary sources of marijuana entering the United States. By 1986, Jamaica, with Belize, Mexico, and Colombia, was listed among the four Caribbean Basin territories that supplied 90 percent of all the marijuana imported into the United States (Maingot 1989, 1994; McDonald 1988; Executive Office of the President 1998; Stone 1991). The INCSR currently designates Jamaica as a major transit point for cocaine entering the United States from South America. U.S. customs also notes that Jamaica is the embarkation point of the largest number of passengers arrested with drugs at U.S. airports. In addition, the Immigration and Naturalization Service and the Drug Enforcement Administration (n.d.) allege that Jamaican drug gangs (termed *posses*) are involved in criminal activities within the United States. Immigration and Naturalization Service statistics indicate that the island is one of the top ten countries for illegal immigrants and fifth for aliens deported from the United States. Consequently, Jamaica, the largest English-speaking Caribbean island, is an excellent case for examining the feasibility of U.S. drug policy assumptions about achieving antidrug targets.

JAMAICA'S SOCIAL, ECONOMIC, AND POLITICAL ENVIRONMENT

Crime trends can be seen as reflectors of social problems within a society. Crime and violence in Jamaica have become of increasing concern both internally and externally. The perception of Jamaica as violent is evident in media reports while the internal reality is reflected in the island's homicides, violent crime rates, and gun-related incidents. These, along with fear of crime, are escalating, and social unrest is occurring more frequently. The consequences for the island have been, and continue to be, devastating, with tourism, the primary foreign exchange earner, being most vulnerable.[2] Because this industry is vulnerable to crime and U.S. State Department travel advisories, violence has significant repercussions on Jamaica's social, economic, and political environments.

LAW ENFORCEMENT AND POLITICAL EXPLANATIONS FOR JAMAICA'S CRIME RATE

The growth of violence is considered the most dramatic manifestation of a decline in Jamaica's social environment. Over the years, a number of Jamaican commissions, councils, task forces, and reports have had the country's crime and violence as their focus.

The Wolfe Report (Wolfe 1993) emerged from public concern over violent upsurges throughout Jamaica between 1991 and 1992. It was constituted to advise on appropriate strategies consistent with the pursuit of justice in the maintenance of law and order (p. 99). The Wolfe Report identified fifteen factors classifiable as social, economic, political, psychological, and administrative that contribute to Jamaica's crime situation. These include problems with the security forces, intolerable and inhumane prison conditions, and a high percentage of foreign female prisoners convicted of drug felonies.

The Wolfe Report recommended implementing recommendations from previous task forces to ameliorate the causes of crime.

CRIME IN JAMAICA

No single factor can adequately account for increased violence in Jamaica. Harriott (1996) noted that Jamaica has become a highly criminogenic society characterized by, among other factors, pervasive criminality that manifests as "disregard for law across all social classes and a developed well-integrated underground economy" (p. 79). Although the violence has changed qualitatively, it has become central, institutionalized, and embedded in different aspects of the national life (Harriott 1996, 80). In the past, political violence and social and economic arrangements were often profiled as possible causes.[3] Violence in Jamaica was of two basic types: geographical and political (Gay and Marquart 1993). The first existed between residents of communities of the corporate areas of Kingston and St. Andrew that differed politically. The second centered on election or other political-party–related concerns.

POLITICAL ENVIRONMENT

Academics and journalists have long documented an intricate connection between politics and violence in Jamaica. Allegedly, politicians imported and distributed guns into poverty-stricken garrison communities to intimidate and coerce community members into party alliance. Several incidents reinforce this belief. These include poignant examples of Jamaican politicians who over the years have attended events such as funerals of individuals of questionable character. These events have generated much controversy within the Jamaican society.

The National Committee on Political Tribalism (Ministry of National Security and Justice 1997) was established "to consider and recommend practical steps to reduce Jamaica's political tensions and violence" (p. 2). Political tribalism, as defined by Blackman (1992), refers to adherence to a political party based on emotional commitment and irrespective of any policy-related or ideological considerations. A manifestation of political tribalism is the use of violence in political activities. The Tribalism Report reiterated the findings of the Wolfe Report and also noted that the high inflow of guns from the United States contributes to Jamaica's crime problems.

In the past, political tribalism and the culture of violence were used to explain increases in Jamaica's crime and violence. Several sources now posit that trade in guns and hard drugs have replaced political tribalism as primary causes of Jamaica's crime (Gunst 1988; Small 1995; Stone 1991). Political and law enforcement personnel attribute current resurgence in Jamaica's violent crime to two main phenomena: deportations from America and "new levels of criminality spurred by international dimensions . . . dedicated to overwhelm our security forces and any institutions which stand in their way" (Crime the target 2001).

DEPORTATION

In 1998, the first full year after implementation of legislation to effect expedited deportation, more than 170,000 individuals were deported from the United States—up from 69,226 in 1996 and 1,000 in 1986. Of the 171,154 deportations in 1998, 56,011 had criminal convictions, with 47 percent having drug convictions (U.S. Department of Justice n.d.-a, n.d.-b). Most countries to which individuals are deported evince underdevelopment, deteriorating economy, and high levels of unemployment.

In 1998, U.S. deportations increased 85 percent over the 1994 totals, but the total proportion of criminals dropped from 66 percent in 1994 to 32.5 percent in 1998. Between 1990 and 1998, more than 12,000 persons were deported to Jamaica, with 71 percent or 8,626 arriving from the United States. Of this number, only 11 percent or 989 were illegal residents. Although criminals comprised only 32.5 percent of persons deported from the United States in 1998, approximately 77 percent of the 1,483 Jamaicans deported from the United States had criminal convictions. Only 16 percent (239 persons) were categorized as illegal aliens; the remainder had criminal convictions, with 49 percent (724 persons) convicted for possession of illegal drugs and 7 percent (116 persons) for illegal possession of firearms. Other categories of offences include robbery, wounding and assault, murder/manslaughter, rape and indecent assault, kidnapping, and money laundering.

Reports consistently cite deportees' contribution to violent crimes in Jamaica. Official sources note that these individuals return with a bag of tricks learned in the United States. Justification for attributing increasing violence to deportees is that current incidents such as carjacking, extortions, dismemberment, and drive-by shootings are not typical of earlier activities. Instead, these acts are part of U.S. drug-related activities and the emergence of American-style violent crime gangs.

A correlation between Jamaican crime trends and deportations indicates that major crimes, especially homicides, rapes, carnal abuse, robberies, and gun-related incidents, have increased concurrently with the commencement of mass deportations to Jamaica (Jamaica Constabulary Force 1996, 1997, 1998a, 1998b, 1999, 2000). Reports of deportee involvement in the Jamaican crime scene published by the *Jamaica Gleaner Online* for 21 June 1999 (Nation at risk 1999) and repeated on 29 June 1999 (Monitoring deportees 1999) assert that from June 1997 to January 1999, deportees were implicated in 600 murders, 1,700 armed robberies, 900 rapes, 150 shootouts with the police, 200 cases of extortion, 3 cases of murdering witnesses, and 10 cases of arson. It is important to note, however, that without empirical studies, the language used says that deportees are "implicated" rather than "responsible for" these crimes.

GUNS

The international world was recently privy to scenes of gunmen engaging Jamaican police in gun-fire.[4] The entry of guns into Jamaican society is a primary factor in the increase in violence. Between 1995 and 1999, guns were used in approximately 65 percent of all homicides, 50 percent of all robberies, and 22 percent of rape/carnal abuse. Customs and the police have seized many caches of guns, with semiautomatic and submachine weapons now replacing revolvers (Edwards 1999). Of the confiscations by the Contraband Enforcement Team, all but one piece was loaded in a United States port (Edwards 1999, 30).

The Jamaican police are concerned with the number of illegal guns because many have strong drug links. Thus, guns entering the region from the United States have been a contentious issue between Caribbean countries and the United States. However, the Bush administration reiterated its opposition to the 2001 United Nations draft accord on the international sale of small arms, warning that it might constrain the legitimate weapons trade and infringe on the right of American citizens to bear arms (Lynch 2001). Drug felons transported to a smaller geographical area, with their gun and drug gang rivalries, have consequences for the social, economic, and political environment. The result is a diversion of resources from areas such as health and education as they make demands on criminal justice resources. The number of riots that have occurred within Jamaica during the past three years suggests that this phenomenon has become the Jamaican response to many situations. Upheavals have historically been associated with the urban poor and disaffected, but recent disturbances have permeated the entire island. Stone (1986) and Harriott (1996) have noted that when massive behavior changes occur in a society during a short time period, there is usually a convergence of factors causing the change, not just one factor.

CHANGES IN THE JAMAICAN DRUG SCENE

The above discussion indicates that the underlying assumptions about the domestic conditions at drug source or in transit zones are incorrect. Of significance, however, is that increased violence, corruption, and gun crimes are currently being observed in the Caribbean region. The Jamaican drug scene exhibits changes consistent with the displacement hypothesis. Jamaica Constabulary Force statistics for the period from 1990 to 1999 show an increase in the volume of drugs transiting the island. These changes include resurgence in the growth of ganja, a shift from marijuana to cocaine, an increase in the volume of cocaine, the spread of drug activities throughout the island, and increased involvement of Colombians in the Jamaican drug scene.

RESURGENCE IN GROWTH OF GANJA

Newspaper reports and analyses of narcotics statistics indicate that the amount of ganja seized continues to be high, with 55,869.59 kilograms seized in 2000. In 1998, 22,924.98

kilograms were seized, down from 24,728.74 kilograms in 1997 and a high of 41,262.7 in 1996 (Anderson 2000). On Thursday, 8 February 2001, compressed ganja weighing 2,727.27 kilograms, or 5,999 pounds, was seized in containers at Kingston Wharves. Three days later, law enforcement interdicted another shipment weighing 18,312 pounds. Methods of concealment are diverse. These include agricultural products such as nutmeg and manufactured goods such as textiles.

The 1999 INCSR reiterates that the United States has provided funding for the Jamaican government's counternarcotics efforts continuously since 1987 and "has provided more counter-narcotics assistance to Jamaica than to any other Caribbean country" (http://www.state.gov/www/global/narcotics_law/1999_narc_report/carib99_part3.html). Citing marijuana shipments leaving Jamaican ports for the United States in commercial cargo, the INCSR was critical of security at Jamaican ports. However, the United States has reduced eradication funding to the island. The U.S. government is reducing its funding of Jamaica's marijuana eradication program in the hope that the Jamaican government will take up the slack (Williams 2000b). In 1999, the Jamaican government agreed to begin paying half of the marijuana cutters' salaries beginning in June 2000 and their full salaries beginning in June 2001. The preferred mode of eradication for the United States is aerial spraying of herbicide. Citing environmental concerns, Jamaica refuses to use this method. Instead, police and military personnel manually eradicate crops. The military have recently been redeployed to the prisons because of labor problems with the prison officers, leaving the responsibility to the police who lack resources and are generally overwhelmed by other domestic crime concerns. With Jamaica's lack of resources to police the harbors and ports (Poor parish with a marvelous serenity 2000), the island becomes an attractive arena in which to conduct illicit narcotic activities. There is now an increase in the quantity of cocaine transiting the island, along with the observed presence and heightened activities of Colombians in Jamaica.

INCREASE IN VOLUME OF COCAINE

The 2000 INCSR, released in March 2001, reveals that the amount of cocaine transiting Jamaica to the United States has quadrupled compared to the same period in 1999, making Jamaica the leading transshipment point in the Caribbean (Ja holds cocaine ranking 1999). The Port Security Corp. acknowledges that attempts to smuggle cocaine through the ports have increased. This is confirmed by Jamaica Constabulary Force statistics on narcotic drugs seized and destroyed that reveal that cocaine seizures tripled between 1996 and 1998. Information is that 1,143.91 kilograms of cocaine were seized in 1998. By comparison, 2,444.46 kilograms were seized between January and 9 December 1999, an increase of 1,300.55 kilograms. In 2000, 1,624.4 kilograms were seized, and 517.99 kilograms were seized up to 30 June 2001.[5]

Factors facilitating this change include lack of resources to police the coastline and drug traffickers' use of technology. Other reasons are that shipment of ganja involves more skill, and cocaine is an easier drug to transship because it has less weight and more value. Law enforcement officials attribute these changes to the dynamism of the trade wherein larger quantities of cocaine are easier to move using body carriers (Jones 1999; INCSR 1999) who are primarily women. Women's involvement in the drug trade and the resulting consequences reinforce the label *feminization of the drug trade* and the reality that the war on drugs has become a war against women. For example, a 14 May 2001 article in the *Jamaica Gleaner Online* (Roxborough 2001) reports that Jamaican women are increasingly being arrested in other jurisdictions for drug-related offences. The number of Jamaican women in British prisons increased from 100 to more than 400 in three years, and between April 1999 and March 2000, 65 percent of the 450 people arrested at British airports for trafficking cocaine came off flights from Jamaica.

Another noticeable change in the Jamaican drug scene is the concentration of cocaine activities in eastern parishes such as the coasts of Portland and St. Thomas. However, lack of resources poses a grave danger as smugglers being pursued by the U.S. Coast Guard under the Shiprider Agreement often unload their cargo. While reports indicate increasing victimization of individuals who have allegedly found this unloaded cargo, very little cooperation is given to the police in their efforts to address the issue (Williams 2000c).

INCREASED PRESENCE OF COLOMBIANS

During the past few years, local and U.S. drug enforcement agents have established that Jamaica is being used as a transshipment point for narcotics and that there is a direct drug link among Jamaicans, Bahamians, and Colombians for this purpose (see the 1999 INCSR). Some Jamaican narcotics officers refer to these forged linkages as the JBC[6] connection wherein Jamaicans provide the routes previously established to traffic ganja, the Bahamians provide navigational services, and the Colombians provide the drugs.

Media reports (Williams 2000a), as well as the INCSR, now indicate increased activities and the presence of Colombians operating in Jamaica. A recent article by the Caribbean News Agency, published in the *Jamaica Gleaner Online* (Sinclair 1999b), cites U.S. State Department sources saying that Colombian drug traffickers have infiltrated many of the Eastern Caribbean nations and have established the services of regional organizations to move drugs in the region. A three-year investigation dubbed White Seas, an initiative of the United States, Canada, Jamaica, and the Bahamas, provided additional evidence of Colombian activities in the region. This investigation revealed that drugs were transported via speedboats from Jamaica and the Bahamas into Miami for distribution in American and Canadian cities (U.S., Canada, Jamaica, Bahamas smash drug ring 2001).

An insider assessment of the cocaine subculture titled "Cocaine Threatening the Nation," published in the *Jamaica Gleaner Online* on 23 January 2000, reiterates the growing importance of Jamaica as a strategic transshipment point in the Colombian cocaine trade and suggests that it is more than a question of geography. Instead, factors include the relative ease with which the traffickers are able to carry out their activities.

The report further explains that heightened surveillance by the U.S. drug enforcement authorities and the local police appears to have had little impact on the trafficking. Colombians gain entry to the island in numerous ways (Sinclair 1999a); consequently, more Colombian nationals may be operating in Jamaica than official estimates indicate.

Colombians are also implicated in increases in gang/turf war, corruption,[7] gun crimes, and stockpiling of cocaine. According to Williams (2000a), increases in gang/turf war in the inner city of Kingston are the result of Colombians operating in Jamaica who want to reduce the number of individuals with whom they deal. Similarly, Professor Don Robotham (2001), in a commentary about the July 2001 West Kingston Affair, noted that the event should not be viewed solely through a domestic political lens. He asserted that no politician or political party is in the position of providing the caliber of guns and ammunitions evident in West Kingston. Consequently, current political instabilities are different from earlier ideological ones. Robotham asserted that sections of West Kingston have become an axis for the international drug trade between Colombia and the rest of the hemisphere. Jamaican media increasingly report activities and influences of Colombians on the Jamaican drug scene.[8] Consequently, though couched in diplomatic terms, the prime minister's statement (Crime the target 2001) on the announcement of the West Kingston Inquiry about "new levels of criminality spurred by international dimensions" is very informative.

Another consequence attributed to the presence of Colombians is the stockpiling of cocaine. According to Jamaican intelligence sources, Colombian drug traffickers bring cocaine to Jamaica to be stockpiled. The cocaine arrives in bulk and leaves in smaller shipments for other places, such as the Bahamas (Jamaica holds cocaine ranking 1999). Colombians are also linked with cruise shipping, especially in tourist areas (Robotham 1999a, 1999b), the potential economic repercussions of which are significant because tourism is vulnerable to U.S. State Department activities and advisories.

Jamaica's involvement in the drug trade has created a dual effect. On one hand, the creation of armed gangs fosters insecurity within the country. On the other hand, these participants become the heroes of the dispossessed youth in their communities. At a minimum, the drug situation has consequences for the policy environment and especially for law enforcement (Thwaites 1999).

An analysis of Colombia's drug situation and the operation of cartels indicates that the operation of Colombians in Jamaica could have consequences for law enforcement and policy implementation (Thwaites 2000). Thachuk (1997) described the activities of Colombian drug traffickers in Colombia as *plomo o' plata*. The English translation of this phrase, "silver or the bullet," gives an indication of the dangers of Colombian drug traffickers to Jamaican society. These include increased drug usage with an attendant rise in addiction and a growth in the incidence of irrational, violent crime that has the potential to undermine and corrupt the government. Recent allegations are that some members of the police force have succumbed to corruption.[9]

While acknowledging that "Jamaica's counter narcotics efforts have taken place against a backdrop of severe resource constraints caused by a continuing recession," the 2000 INCSR derides Jamaica, noting that increased trafficking "indicates the need for the GOJ to intensify and focus its law enforcement efforts and to enhance its international co-operation." Clearly, the United States sees the increased volume of drug trafficking to be a shortcoming of Jamaican initiatives rather than the result of its drug policy. Intensification of law enforcement could prove a problem. The island's law enforcement practices are currently under international scrutiny. Amnesty International (2001) issued a scathing report of law enforcement in Jamaica titled *Jamaica: Killings and Violence by Police. How Many More Victims?* that documents gross abuses by law enforcement personnel.

SUMMARY/ CONCLUSION

U.S.-funded antidrug initiatives in Colombia result in compensating behavior such as displacement activities. Observed changes in Jamaica include an increase in crime and violence, a worsening of the formal economy, increased presence of Colombian nationals, and an increase in the amount of drugs transiting the island. These are contrary to the drug policy assumptions respecting source countries' capabilities and domestic conditions. Consequently, the premises underlying the supply reduction policy are incorrect. More important, attempts at conforming to U.S.-imposed targets lead to undue costs for these societies. Many cannot afford to expend the level of resources required to sustain antidrug initiatives.

While domestic concerns necessitate a focus on wealth creation or poverty alleviation, a disproportionate antidrug budget diverts resources from said programs, thereby increasing the likelihood of negative economic growth. A depressed or stagnant economy increases the likelihood that the mass of unemployed and underemployed population will engage in illegal drug trade. Moreover, large-scale legal and illegal immigration are the most prominent symptoms of economic instability in the Caribbean. These thwart the goals of reducing illegal immigration or severing drugs at the source.

Policy impositions are having consequences for the entire Caribbean region. Problems are displaced into areas where the resources for addressing drug issues are minimal, with some countries being disproportionately affected. Jamaica, already lacking in resources, is in for a rough time.[10] For example, recent newspaper headlines such as "Jamaica Tops Region in Cocaine Transshipment" (Associated Press 2001) and "This Is Bigger than Us: Cops Helpless as Drug Planes Land at Airport" (http://www.jamaica-gleaner.com/gleaner/20010325/lead/lead1.html) indicate some of the consequences for Jamaica. Simultaneously, it appears that the Colombian crackdown has accelerated the dispersion of drug trafficking activities throughout the Caribbean region. Its major consequence, however, may be the transformation of Jamaica's political tribalism into a narco-political tribalism. Cumulatively, both immigration and drug policies allow deported persons to continue their drug- and gun-related activities. Since these changes were observed before full implementation of Plan Colombia, it is reasonable to conclude that further displacement will occur. Similarly, displacement of U.S. antidrug initiatives may be exacerbated by the refusal to implement more restrictive gun policies.

Not only have the U.S. policies failed to achieve their goals; they have had adverse consequences for some countries. Yet fear of repercussions such as decertification limits governmental responses to domestic drug control initiatives. Consequently, Caribbean countries are not at liberty to implement best practices from other jurisdictions or implement policies that are not endorsed by the United States. This indicates that the conceptualization of drug war casualties needs to be broadened.

Notes

1. The Colombian government has developed a comprehensive, integrated strategy called Plan Colombia to address Colombia's drug and interrelated social and economic troubles. Plan Colombia focuses on five strategic issues: (1) the peace process, (2) the Colombian economy, (3) the counterdrug strategy, (4) the reform of the justice system and the protection of human rights, and (5) democratization and social development (Executive Office of the President 2001, 14). The program is expected to cost $7.5 billion, with $1.6 billion proposed U.S. support over the fiscal years 2000 and 2001. This represents an increase of $1.3 billion from the previous $330 million (Strategy FY 2001 Budget, 14-22). As stated therein,

> Since there is no single solution to Colombia's difficulty . . . it is in the national interest of the United States to stem the flow of illegal drugs and to promote stability and strengthen democracy in Colombia and the Andean region. (P. 16)

Thus, the U.S. contribution to Plan Colombia has five components centered on reducing the supply of Colombian drugs to the United States.

2. For example, after the April 1999 incident, visitor arrivals decreased, requiring an infusion of U.S.$1.8 million to help bolster Jamaica's international image (Virtue 1999). The same effects were noticed after the recent West Kingston events of 7-10 July 2001.

3. Chuck (1999) suggested that the decline in the economy accounts for the cycle of brutality that has overtaken the society. He suggests that the worsening economy has affected the quality of life and promoted the decline of civility and decency. In fact, nowhere is it more dramatically displayed than in the inner cities. The rising tension, gang warfare, protection money, lack of opportunities and deteriorating conditions can all be traced to an economy derailed and heading for disaster.

4. This was the perception of Father Howard Rochester, then at St. Richard's Catholic Church, Red Hills, who also became a casualty of this siege when he was found murdered in October 2000. Examples of this siege include the Tivoli Gardens incident of May 1997, so named because the Jamaican security forces and residents of Tivoli Gardens in West Kingston engaged in what the press labeled a "battle." Between 19 and 21 April 1999, the island was again under siege as Jamaicans engaged in mass demonstrations or as both the local and international press labeled it, "rioted" in response to a 30 percent increase in the price of petrol. Again in June of 1999, Kingston experienced a spate of killings with approximately sixty-six people killed in seventeen days. The Mountain View incident, so named because residents of the area, in solidarity with the gunmen, declared the area off limits to police, happened in April 2000. Gunmen engaged the police in continual gun battle, often forcing them into retreat. Criminal justice statistics for 2000 reveal that seventy people were murdered in the first twenty-five days of April 2000, fifty-six of them in the Kingston Metropolitan region. In the latest incident, twenty-five people were killed during the period of 7-10 July 2001.

5. See Jamaica holds cocaine ranking (1999) regarding information on the seizure of a Colombian boat with 700 kilograms of cocaine. This amount increases the seizures to 1,217.99 kilograms for this period.

6. JBC is also the acronym for the now defunct Jamaica Broadcasting Corporation.

7. For example, the *Jamaica Daily Gleaner* of 27 October 2000 reported that prison warders and police officers were being questioned to ascertain who aided and abetted two Colombians who were released from the correctional facility where they were being held.

8. A poignant story from the *Jamaica Gleaner Online* for Thursday, 19 July 2001 titled "Mystery Surrounds Theft of Drug Boat from Police Custody" (2001) reports that

> Colombian drug traffickers have been using a seized boat they stole from police custody last month to continue their trade in Jamaican territorial waters.... But local law enforcers are unable to catch up with the drug smugglers [because] their marine vehicles are no match for the twin-engine boats used by the traffickers.

The boat was seized in April with twenty-four cocaine packets weighing approximately 700 kilograms (1,540 pounds) with a Jamaican street value of $195 million.

9. In January 1998, Police Commissioner Francis Forbes transferred 56 of the 127 police personnel from Portland because some were suspected to have been involved in cocaine trafficking in the parish.

10. This is confirmed by activities during 7-10 July 2001, now referred to as the West Kingston Affairs, when media coverage showed gunmen engaging the Jamaican police in three days of cross fire.

References

Amnesty International. 2001. Jamaica: Killings and violence by police. How many more victims? *Jamaica Gleaner Online*, 4 October. Available from http://www.jamaica-gleaner.com/pages/amnesty/full/index.html.

Anderson, Omar. 2000. Less ganja, more cocaine in Jamaica. *Jamaica Gleaner Online*, 5 March. Retrieved from http://www.jamaica-gleaner.com/gleaner/20000305/index.html.

Arganaras, Fernando Garcia. 1997. Harm reduction at the supply side of the drug war: The case of Bolivia. In *Harm reduction: A new direction for drug policies and programs*, edited by Patricia G. Erickson, Diane M. Riley, Yuet W. Cheung, and Patrick A. O'Hare. Toronto, Canada: University of Toronto Press.

Associated Press. 2001. Jamaica tops region in cocaine transshipment. *Jamaica Gleaner Online*, 12 March. Retrieved from http://www.jamaica-gleaner.com/gleaner/20010312/news/news3.html.

Blackman, Kenneth. 1992. Jamaica: Drugs, politics and poverty blamed for wave of violence. *Interpress Service*, 6 March.

Bureau of Western Hemispheric Fact Sheet, Andean Regional Initiative. 2001. Retrieved 16 May from http://www. state.gov/e/rls/index.cfm?docid= 2980 [2001-09-18].

Chuck, Delroy. 1999. Vortex of decline. *Jamaica Gleaner Online*, 30 June. Retrieved from http://www.go-jamaica. com/gleaner/19990630/.

Cocaine threatening the nation. 2000. *Jamaica Gleaner Online*, 23 January. Available from http://www.go-jamaica.com.

Craig, Richard B. 1987. Illicit drug traffic: Implications for South American source countries. *Journal of Intra-American Studies and World Affairs* 29 (2): 1-34.

Crime the target—PM announces West Kingston inquiry. 2001. *Jamaica Gleaner Online*, 16 July. Retrieved from http://www.jamaica-gleaner. com/gleaner/20010716/lead/ lead2.html.

Drug Enforcement Administration. n.d. *The Jamaican posse*. Intelligence bulletin 90 (2). New York: New York Field Division, Unified Intelligence Division.

Edwards, D. T. 1999. The prevalence of firearm related offenses in Jamaica and implications for national security. M.Sc. diss., Royal Military College of Science, Department of Defense, Management and Security Analysis, Cranfield Security Centre, Shrivenham, UK.

Executive Office of the President, United States, Office of National Drug Control Policy. 1997. *National drug control strategy*. Retrieved from http://www. whitehousedrugpolicy.gov/publications/ policy/ndcs01/index.html.

———. 1998. *National drug control strategy*. Retrieved from http://www. whitehousedrugpolicy.gov/publications/ policy/ndcs01/index.html.

———. 1999. *National drug control strategy*. Retrieved from http://www. whitehousedrugpolicy.gov/publications/ policy/ndcs01/index.html.

———. 2000. *National drug control strategy*. Retrieved from http://www. whitehousedrugpolicy.gov/publications/ policy/ndcs01/index.html.

———. 2001. *National drug control strategy*. Retrieved from http://www. whitehousedrugpolicy.gov/publications/ policy/ndcs01/index.html.

Gabor, Thomas. 1981. The crime displacement hypothesis: An empirical examination. *Crime & Delinquency* 27:390-404.

Gay, Bruce W., and James M. Marquart. 1993. Jamaican posses: A new form of organized crime. *Journal of Crime and Justice* 16 (2): 139-70.

Gunst, Laurie. 1988. *Born fi dead*. New York: Holt.

Harriott, Anthony. 1996. The changing social organization of crime and criminals in Jamaica. *Caribbean Quarterly* 42 (2/3): 61-81.

Ja holds cocaine ranking. 1999. *Jamaica Gleaner Online*, 19 October. Retrieved from http://www.jamaica-gleaner. com/gleaner/19991019/f2.html.

Jamaica Constabulary Force. 1996. *Annual report*. Kingston, Jamaica: Government Printing Office.

———. 1997. *Annual report*. Kingston, Jamaica: Government Printing Office.

———. 1998a. *Annual report*. Kingston, Jamaica: Government Printing Office.

———. 1998b. [Crime statistics]. Unpublished raw data.

———. 1999. [Crime statistics]. Unpublished raw data.

————. 2000. [Crime statistics]. Unpublished raw data.

Jamaica holds cocaine ranking. 1999. *Jamaica Gleaner Online*, 19 October. Retrieved from http://www.jamaica-gleaner.com/gleaner/19991019/index.html.

Jones, Karen. 1999. Narcotic strategy yields result. *Jamaica Gleaner Online*, 15 June. Retrieved from http://www.jamaica-gleaner.com/gleaner/19990615/index.html.

Lynch, Colum. 2001. U.S. fights UN accord to fight small arms. *Washington Post*, 10 July, A01. Retrieved from http://www.washingtonpost.com/wp-dyn/world/A38049-2001Jul9.html.

Maingot, Anthony. 1989. The drug menace to the Caribbean. *The World and I* (July): 128-35.

————. 1994. *The United States and the Caribbean*. Boulder, CO: Westview.

McDonald, Scott B. 1988. *Dancing on a volcano: The Latin American drug trade*. New York: Praeger.

Ministry of National Security and Justice. 1997. *Report of the National Committee on Political Tribalism*. Kingston, Jamaica: Government Printing Office.

Monitoring deportees. 1999. *Jamaica Gleaner Online*, 29 June. Retrieved from http//:www.jamaica-gleaner.com/19990629.

Mystery surrounds theft of drug boat from police custody. 2001. *Jamaica Gleaner Online*, 19 July. Retrieved from http://www.jamaica-gleaner.com/gleaner/20010719/lead/lead4.html.

Nation at risk. 1999. *Jamaica Gleaner Online*, 21 June. Retrieved from http//:www.jamaica-gleaner.com/19990621.

Office of National Drug Control Policy. 1998. *Performance measures of effectiveness*. Washington, DC: Executive Office of the President, Office of National Drug Control Policy.

————. 2000. *Performance measures of effectiveness*. Washington, DC: Executive Office of the President, Office of National Drug Control Policy.

Performance Management Evaluation. 2000. Washington, DC: Executive Office of the President, Office of National Drug Control Policy.

Poor parish with a marvelous serenity. 2000. *Jamaica Gleaner Online*, 23 March. Retrieved from http://www.jamaica-gleaner.com/gleaner/20000323/index.html.

Robotham, Don. 1999a. Crime and public policy in Jamaica (part 2). *Jamaica Gleaner Online*, 17 August. Retrieved from http://www.jamaica-gleaner.com/gleaner/19990817/cleisure/index.html.

————. 1999b. Roots of crime (2). *Jamaica Gleaner Online*, 19 August. Retrieved from http://www.jamaica-gleaner.com/gleaner/19990819/cleisure/index.html.

————. 2001. The cocaine connection. *Jamaica Gleaner Online*, 17 July. Retrieved from http://www.jamaica-gleaner.com/gleaner/20010717/cleisure/cleisure2.html.

Roxborough, Pat. 2001. J'cans crowd UK prisons—British team coming to probe reasons local women smuggle drugs. Jamaica Gleaner Online, 14 May. Retrieved from http://www.jamaica-gleaner.com/gleaner/20010514/lead/lead2.html.

Sinclair, Glenroy. 1999a. Colombians held in hotel. *Jamaica Daily Gleaner*, 16 July.

————. 1999b. U.S. finds most drugs on passengers from Jamaica. *Jamaica Gleaner Online*, 21 September. Retrieved from http://www.jamaica-gleaner.com/gleaner/19990921/f2.html.

Small, Geoff. 1995. *Ruthless: The global rise of the yardies*. London: Warner Books.

Smith, Peter. 1992. The political economy of drugs: Conceptual issues and policy options. In *Drug policy in the Americas*, edited by Peter Smith. Boulder, CO: Westview.

Stone, Carl. 1986. *Class, state and democracy in Jamaica*. New York: Praeger.

———. 1991. Hard drug use in a black island society. *Caribbean Affairs* 4 (2): 142-61.

Thachuk, K. 1997. Plomo o plata: Politics, corruption and drug policy in Colombia. Ph.D. thesis, Simon Fraser University, Burnaby, British Colombia, Canada.

Thwaites, Daniel. 1999. The usual suspect. *Jamaica Gleaner Online*, 16 July. Retrieved from http://www.jamaica-gleaner.com/gleaner/19990716/index.html.

———. 2000. How low can we go? *Jamaica Gleaner Online*, 20 October. Retrieved from http://www.jamaica-gleaner.com/gleaner/20001020/cleisure/cleisure4.html.

U.S., Canada, Jamaica, Bahamas smash drug ring. 2001. Retrieved from http://www.wjin.net/html/news/7197.htm/ 2/5/01.

U.S. Department of Justice, Immigration and Naturalization Services. n.d.-a. *Detention and removal fact sheet and statistics*. Retrieved from http://www. ins.usdoj.gov/graphics/publicaffairs/factsheets/Deten.pdf 2000-12-13.

———. n.d.-b. *Statistics*. Retrieved from http://www.ins.usdoj.gov/graphics/aboutins/statistics/Illegals.htm 2001-08-01.

Virtue, Erica. 1999. Gas riots leave long-term damage. *Jamaica Gleaner Online*, 14 November. Retrieved from http://www.go-jamaica.com/gleaner/19991114/f1.html.

White House, Office of the Press Secretary. 2000. Press release on Colombia assistance package. Grand Canyon, AZ: Office of the Press Spokesman.

Williams, Lloyd. 2000a. Colombians take control of local cocaine trade. *Jamaica Gleaner Online*, 23 January. Retrieved from http://www.jamaica-gleaner.com/gleaner/20000123/index.html.

———. 2000b. US$ ganja cut-back. *Jamaica Gleaner Online*, 13 March. Available from http://www.jamaica-gleaner.com.

———. 2000c. Washed up cocaine, gunman and violence. *Jamaica Gleaner Online*, 24 January. Retrieved from http://www.jamaica-gleaner.com/gleaner/20000124/index.html.

Wolfe, L. 1993. *Report of the National Task Force on Crime*. Kingston, Jamaica: Government Printing Office.

ANNALS, *AAPSS*, **582**, July 2002

Mexico's War on Drugs:
No Margin for Maneuver

By JORGE CHABAT

ABSTRACT: Illegal drugs threaten the Mexican governance because of the corruption they generate. The Mexican government has been fighting this threat for years in a context of institutional weakness and strong pressures from the United States. The fact that Mexico is a natural supplier of illegal drugs to the biggest market in the world, the United States, puts the Mexican government in a very complex situation with no alternatives other than to continue fighting drugs with very limited institutional and human resources. In this process, Mexico has no margin for maneuver to change the parameters of the war on drugs.

Jorge Chabat is an associate professor in the Department of International Studies at the Center for Research and Teaching in Economics in Mexico City. He is an expert on U.S.-Mexican relations, drug trafficking, and national security issues. He has edited, with John Bailey, the book Transnational Crime and Public Security: Challenges to Mexico and the United States *(2002, University of California, San Diego). He is a regular political commentator for Mexican newspapers and television.*

I LLEGAL drugs affect Mexico in terms of both consumption and traffic. However, although drug consumption has increased in Mexico during recent years, it is far from being a serious social problem, and the levels remain very low compared to those of industrialized countries. Therefore, traffic is the main problem in Mexico because of the corruption it generates. And since the traffic of illicit drugs is highly motivated by the demands that exist in consumer countries, the problem in Mexico is influenced in an important measure by the demand in the United States. At the same time, it is U.S. pressure on Mexico that propels a very aggressive drug control policy in Mexico. The combination of U.S. pressure and the role of Mexico as a major point of transit of drugs entering the United States has generated serious tension in Mexican law enforcement institutions. Since the Mexican government is not able to modify these parameters, it has very little margin for maneuver in the war on drugs, and it seems confined to fight a very costly war that endangers the Mexican transition to democracy.

Mexico has been fighting illegal drugs for a century. In 1912, Mexico supported the Hague International Opium Convention, and during the following years, the Mexican government prohibited trade of the main illegal drugs: opium, cocaine, and marijuana. During the first three decades of the twentieth century, a pattern emerged: Mexico became a producer of heroin and marijuana as well as a provider to the United States of these drugs. At the same time, there were increasing pressures from the American government on its southern neighbor to develop a more effective strategy against drugs. Even before drug trafficking was a national security issue in Mexico, there were some scandals of drug corruption in the 1930s, like the resignation of the minister of the interior, Carlos Riva Palacio, in 1931 (Walker 1981).

Notwithstanding, drug trafficking was not an important topic on the Mexican domestic or international agenda until the 1980s. Although there have been addicts since the 1920s when it was possible to find opium smoking rooms in Mexicali on the border with the United States, it has not been a social problem of important dimensions, as in the United States. During the 1940s and 1950s, the Mexican government developed a punitive approach toward illegal drugs, increasing the penalties for drug traffickers and signing all international agreements to fight the traffic of illicit drugs. The Mexican counterdrug efforts proved to be efficient during the 1970s when Operation Condor was implemented as a result of the pressure by the Nixon administration in 1969. The success achieved by the Mexican government in the eradication of marijuana and opium were used by the U.S. government as an example of what a country can do about fighting drugs if there is political will. However, the antidrug effort deteriorated during the 1980s. Mexico appeared again as an important supplier of marijuana and heroin to the United

States and emerged as a point of transit for the cocaine coming from South America. The new role of Mexico in the international chain of drug trafficking provoked some friction with the United States, aggravated by the traditional anti-U.S. feeling existing in part of the Mexican population. The assassination of the Drug Enforcement Administration (DEA) agent Enrique Camarena in Mexico in 1985, with the complicity of the Mexican Federal Police, was only the tip of the iceberg of a growing problem that was affecting Mexican domestic politics as well as Mexico's foreign relations. Since then, drug trafficking has become a national security problem because of its impact on violence and corruption. At the same time, consumption of illicit drugs emerged as a growing problem with social repercussions. What is the state of the drug problem in Mexico right now? What has the Mexican government done? What are the failures and the limits in this war? And finally, what are Mexico's options?

THE NATURE OF THE PROBLEM

During the second half of the 1980s, Mexico became the source of 70 percent of the marijuana and 25 percent of the heroin imported by the United States, as well as the territory through which 60 percent of the cocaine entering the United States was transported (Chabat 1994). In the 1990s, the situation did not change, except for the fact that Mexican cartels became more powerful, according to DEA sources (U.S. Department of Justice; see also

Constantine 1996). The fact that Mexican drug cartels were more powerful had an impact in terms of the levels of violence and corruption and, probably, in the levels of drug consumption.

According to the DEA, by the end of the 1980s, traffickers from Mexico were able to deliver drugs in the United States, replacing the Colombian drug organization. This tendency was reinforced in the mid-1990s after the arrest of the Cali Cartel leaders. In 1996, DEA Director Thomas A. Constantine denounced the existence of a Mexican drug trafficking federation made up of four major cartels: the Tijuana Organization, the Sonora Cartel, the Juarez Cartel, and the Gulf Group (Constantine 1996). However, during the second half of the 1990s, the Gulf Cartel grew weaker due in part to the arrest of its leader, Juan Garcia Abrego, in 1996. Some analysts have speculated that the decline of the Gulf Cartel was related to the fact that the Salinas administration (1988-1994) protected it, and that this protection vanished with the arrival of the Zedillo administration (1994-2000). It is difficult to prove that assertion, but Garcia Abrego himself declared in testimony during his trial in the United States that his cartel obtained the cocaine it smuggled into the United States from the seizures made by the attorney general's office of other drug cartels. Whatever the reasons for this decline, it was evident that the more powerful cartels at the end of the decade were the Tijuana and the Juarez Cartels. According to

Mexican official sources, the appearance of a drug cartel in the Yucatan peninsula (known as the Cancun Cartel) in the late 1990s was due to the expansion of the Juarez Cartel. In any case, both cartels are well and alive, even when the Juarez Cartel leader apparently died during plastic surgery in July 1997. Independent of the veracity of this version, the Juarez mafia was able to reorganize itself very quickly, and its alleged new leader, Vicente Carrillo Fuentes (brother of Amado Carrillo), has not been captured. In addition, the Tijuana cartel has been operating for many years, and does not show many signs of weakening, despite the death of its leader, Ramon Arellano Felix, and the arrest of his brother, Benjamin, in 2002. This situation was denounced by the U.S. ambassador to Mexico, Jeffrey Davidow, in February 2000, when he said that Mexico had become a world headquarters for the drug trade.

Notwithstanding the growing power of the Mexican drug mafias, there is no evidence that they are involved in other forms of organized crime, like kidnappings or car thefts. The link between drug trafficking and other forms of common criminality is difficult to prove (for this discussion and the case of Mexico, see Bailey and Chabat 2001). However, there is a correlation between the rise in crime rates in Mexico and the strengthening of drug trafficking cartels in the mid-1990s.

In terms of production, the figures for marijuana and opium—the only two illicit crops developed in Mexican territory—have been quite stable during the 1990s. By 2000, Mexico was still an important supplier of both drugs to the United States, even though Mexican production of opium represents less than 2 percent of the world's production. In 2000, according to the U.S. State Department (2001), Mexico was also the point of transit of 55 percent of cocaine entering the United States.

It is difficult to have an exact figure for the money that drug trafficking generates in Mexico, but most of the calculations places it between $6 billion and $15 billion annually,[1] representing between 1 percent and 3 percent of Mexico's GDP. However, taking into consideration the volume of cocaine transported through Mexico as well as the volume of marijuana and heroine produced in the country, it is very feasible to think of a figure of about $3 billion per year. It is also difficult to give a reliable figure of the number of people involved in drug trafficking. However, since the cultivation of both marijuana and opium requires the labor of many peasants, it is not an exaggeration to think of many thousands involved in the production and distribution of these drugs. Notwithstanding, given the population of the country (100 million people), it is difficult to say that drug trafficking generates an important part of the employment in Mexico. Nevertheless, the economic impact is concentrated in a few regions in Central and Northern Mexico, particularly the states of Michoacan, Sinaloa, and Chihuahua.

Regarding consumption, the latest official figure available shows that in 1998, 1.23 percent of the urban population were regular consumers (those who used some illegal drug during the past year), that is, approximately 600,000 people. Even though this figure is very low compared with the figures in the United States, consumption of illegal drugs in Mexico increased 30 percent from 1993 to 1998 (Mexico, Secretaria de Salud 1999). There are several causes for this increase. The process of economic modernization that Mexico has experienced during the past two decades is an important factor to explain the increase in the use of illegal drugs in the main cities of Mexico. However, the fact that during recent years, the drug cartels paid drug smugglers for their services with drugs has contributed to the expansion of Mexican demand for illicit drugs. In any case, it is important to point out that although drug consumption is increasing in Mexico, the main problem with drugs is cultivation and traffic. This characteristic directly determines the interests and options of Mexico vis-à-vis illegal drugs.

THE COSTS OF DRUG TRAFFICKING: VIOLENCE AND CORRUPTION

Although violence has increased during recent years, it remains confined to some regions and basically affects only those who are involved in the business or in law enforcement activities. In this regard, there is no evidence that drug-related violence constitutes a threat to governance in Mexico. Notwithstanding, there are some notorious cases of murders of policemen, journalists, and politicians. Among these cases are the killing of Tijuana Police Chief Federico

Benitez Lopez in April 1994; the assassination of former federal prosecutor Arturo Ochoa Palacio in 1996; the killing of Ernesto Ibarra Santes, the newly named head of federal police operations in Baja California in 1996; and the murder of Baja California State Prosecutor Hodin Gutierrez in 1997. Drug-related violence rose significantly in some cities in Northern Mexico, principally Tijuana and Ciudad Juarez. In 1997, the Mexican authorities reported the disappearance of 100 people in Ciudad Juarez, most of them probably related to drug trafficking. The drug-related violence also reached a prominent journalist, Jesus Blancornelas, *Zeta* newspaper editor, who survived an assassination attempt in November 1997, and the governor of the Mexican state of Chihuahua, Patricio Martínez, who also survived an assassination attempt in February 2001, although in this case the drug connection has not been clearly established. There are also suspicions that drug trafficking was involved in the assassination of Revolutionary Institutional Party (PRI) presidential candidate Luis Donaldo Colosio in 1994 and Cardinal Jesus Posadas Ocampo in 1993, but there is no clear evidence of this link.

Corruption has been present in the Mexican government during the past two decades and has been a source of friction between Mexico and the United States. The most notorious case was that of General Jesus Gutierrez-Rebollo, the head of the National Institute for the Combat of Drugs, arrested in 1997 for collaborating with the Juarez Cartel. There also were cases of corruption in the Salinas and the Zedillo administrations. According to the media, high officers of the Salinas administration were involved with drug trafficking, including Salinas's chief of staff Jose Cordoba and his brother Raul Salinas de Gortari. Some American newspapers suggested that members of Zedillo's cabinet, including the secretary of defense, General Enrique Cervantes, and the private secretary of the president, Liebano Saenz, were linked to drug trafficking. The *New York Times* suggested in February 1997 that the governors of the Mexican states of Sonora and Morelos, Manlio Fabio Beltrones and Jorge Carrillo Olea, were involved in drug trafficking. In February 1998, the *Washington Times* accused Francisco Labastida, at that time secretary of the interior (Gobernacion) and in 2000 presidential candidate of the PRI, of collaborating with drug traffickers when he was governor of the Mexican state of Sinaloa in the late 1980s and early 1990s. In all these cases, there was no legal action against these officials. If these accusations are at least partially true, drug trafficking really is posing a threat to the Mexican state's ability to govern.

One example of the corrupting ability of drug traffickers is the escape from a high-security prison of the Mexican drug lord Joaquin "Chapo" Guzman in January 2001. This event shows the degree of corruption that has pervaded the Mexican government, as was acknowledged by Under Secretary of Public Security Jorge Tello Peon.

Another corrupting influence of drug trafficking is the possible presence of drug money in political campaigns. Although some analysts suggested that there has been some drug financing in the Zedillo campaign and perhaps some other local campaigns, there is no clear evidence of that (see Lupsha 1995). Also, it seems that drug traffickers have no political preference. They try to influence politicians of all parties, not only those belonging to the PRI, which has held the Mexican presidency since 1929 and has dominated the Mexican political system since then.

MEXICAN COUNTERDRUG EFFORTS

During the past decades, the Mexican government has dedicated important economic and human resources to fight drugs. In terms of the combat of the traffic of illicit drugs, the Mexican government has been using the Federal Judicial Police for years, but the results have been quite disappointing. Corruption has made the Mexican police very inefficient. I have already mentioned some examples of drug-related corruption. This is the reason why President Zedillo decided to send the army to fight drug traffickers in the beginning of his administration. Since the 1950s, the Mexican army has been collaborating in the eradication of illicit crops, but it had no responsibility in law enforcement. In that sense, the use of the army to collaborate in the arrest of drug traffickers represents an important change in the Mexican counterdrug efforts.

The effectiveness of the Mexican army in fighting drugs is mixed. The army has been effective in the capture of some drug traffickers, such as "El Güero" Palma in June 1995, but it could not arrest the Juarez Cartel leader Amado Carrillo in 1997, probably because the Mexican drug czar General Gutierrez Rebollo alerted the drug lord. These failures and cases of corruption have fueled criticisms of the army's new role, but the truth is that nobody has been able to show a clear alternative, given the deterioration of the police forces in Mexico. Discussion about the appropriateness of using the army in fighting drug trafficking shows how serious narco-corruption is in Mexico and that no one is immune to it.

There was little variation of seizures and eradication during the 1990s (see U.S. State Department 2000). There was some progress in marijuana and heroin seizures, but not in cocaine. In any case, the general tendency does not allow us to talk about any significant change, despite the efforts announced by the Mexican government and in response to U.S. pressure.

The results of efforts to dismantle criminal organizations is also mixed. Some important drug lords have been arrested, but the cartels continue operating. As has been mentioned, in 1995, the Mexican army captured El Güero Palma, leader of the Sinaloa Cartel. However, the most notorious case was the arrest of Juan Garcia Abrego, leader of the Gulf Cartel, who was deported to the United States in January 1996 because he was a U.S. citizen. Zedillo

also arrested two important members of the Tijuana Cartel as well as a lieutenant to the Gulf Cartel leader. Until May 2000, the Zedillo administration had captured 451 members of drug trafficking organizations. Zedillo also implemented in 1998 the so-called Maxi-proceso, an operation that attacked the Juarez Cartel and that led to the arrest of some businessmen and the prosecution of Mario Villanueva Madrid, governor of the Mexican state of Quintana Roo. This was the first time in modern Mexican history that an acting governor had an arrest order. Unfortunately, it was not enforced because Villanueva escaped some days before the end of his term. He was finally captured in May 2001 by the Fox administration.

Zedillo also arrested, in 2000, other high military officers like General Arturo Acosta Chaparro, a one-star general, and General Francisco Quiros Hermosillo, a three-star general accused of collaborating with the Juarez Cartel. In 1997, General Alfredo Navarro Lara was arrested, accused of having links with the Tijuana Cartel. Also, there were some arrests of police officers, including that of the former director of the Federal Judicial Police, Adrian Carrera Fuentes, who was allowed by the Mexican government to testify in the United States. By May 2000, there were 3,060 law enforcement officers suspended for corruption.

The Fox administration also attacked the drug cartels. In May 2001, the Mexican government arrested Adan Amezcua, one of the leaders of the Colima Cartel, dedicated to the production of methamphetamines. Also, in February 2001, Fox ordered the arrest of all officials in the attorney general's office in the Mexican state of Chihuahua, accused of collaborating with the Juarez Cartel. In April 2001, Fox arrested nineteen members of the Gulf Cartel, including a trafficker known as "El June." In May 2001, as it has been mentioned, Fox also arrested fugitive Mario Villanueva, former governor of Quintana Roo. On 7 June 2001, an important drug lord from the Gulf Cartel, Juan Garza, surrendered himself to U.S. authorities.

During recent years, particularly in the 1990s, the Mexican government has made important institutional and legal reforms to improve the capacity of the Mexican state to fight drugs. Following the Cardinal Posadas assassination in 1993, the Salinas administration created the National Institute for the Combat of Drugs to better coordinate the fight against drug trafficking. In December 1993, the criminal code was reformed to increase the length of sentences for drug traffickers and the number of days they can be maintained in custody. These reforms also facilitate the confiscation and sale of goods belonging to drug traffickers and the government's access to information about drug trafficking. In July 1993, the Mexican government modified the federal fiscal code, establishing reporting for the entry of foreign exchange in amounts of more than U.S.$10,000 into Mexican territory. Since 1990, money laundering has been defined as a felony.

The Ernesto Zedillo administration continued the tendency showed by Salinas de Gortari to improve the indicators in the fight against drugs. Concerning institutional reforms, Zedillo enacted a new law against organized crime in December 1996. This law strengthened the penalties against organized crime and targets criminal association, similar to the Racketeering Influence and Corrupt Organizations (RICO) law in the United States. The new law allowed telephonic interception, protection of witnesses, covert agents, and seizures of goods. To enforce this law, Zedillo created the Special Unit against Organized Crime. Zedillo also established a Special Unit against Money Laundering. In 1997, after the arrest of its director, Zedillo abolished the National Institute for the Combat of Drugs and created the special attorney for Crimes Against Health post inside the attorney general's office. In 1997, the Zedillo administration promoted constitutional reforms to make the fight against crime more efficient. These reforms were approved in March 1999. In August 1998, Zedillo launched the National Crusade against Crime, whose purpose was to modernize the fight against crime. In December of that year, Zedillo created the federal preventive police, which absorbed some other federal police forces, such as the highway police, the fiscal police, and the migration police. In 1999, the Mexican government launched the so-called Operación Sellamiento de la Frontera (Sealing the Border Operation), aimed at stopping drugs before they enter Mexican territory. The Mexican government announced an additional expenditure of around $500 million during two years. This operation dedicated most of the budget to high-tech hardware, including X-ray machines to inspect trucks coming from Central America, high-speed boats, and small surveillance planes. The Zedillo government arrested 63,645 persons, a substantial decline from the Salinas de Gortari administration (more than 100,000 persons).

It is also worth mentioning that the Mexican government has been dedicating important amounts of money to fight drug trafficking during the past decade. In 1991, the amount of money dedicated to fight drug trafficking was about U.S.$100 million. According to nonofficial sources, the amount the Mexican government spent annually in fighting drugs was calculated by the end of 1994 at around $500 million (Drug Strategies 1994). However, this figure could have been affected by the devaluation of the peso in December 1994. In 1997, official sources said that the antidrug budget was around $1 billion.[2] By 1998, the antidrug money represented one-third of the total budget of the attorney general's office.

THE AMERICAN FACTOR: THE CERTIFICATION PROCESS

Since the beginning of the twentieth century, the Mexican counterdrug efforts have been influenced by the United States either in a direct way or through the international agreements in which the American government has played an important role. American pressure increased significantly in the 1970s, paving the way to the successful Operation Condor. However, the pressure became much stronger in the 1980s, especially after Camarena's assassination in 1985. In part as a result of this event, in 1986, the U.S. government implemented the certification process, which established the legal obligation of the U.S. president to inform Congress about the performance of countries involved in the production or transit of drugs in fighting illegal drugs. While full certification has been granted to Mexico every year without exception since 1986, it has been a source of public friction between both countries. It has become almost a ritual every year, in the weeks before the certification, for the Mexican authorities to invoke the defense of sovereignty to condemn this process as unilateral and unfair. And since the certification process measures basically political will and not necessarily final results in terms of real reduction of the flow of drugs, it has been used more as a political instrument than as an effective mechanism to reduce drug trafficking or consumption (see Reuter and Ronfeldt 1992). The elements taken into account to grant certification have provoked the Mexican government to dedicate much of its energy to fulfill these indicators. The criteria for granting certification are (1) a budget dedicated to fight drug trafficking, (2) seizures and eradication of shipments, (3) the number of arrests, (4) legal and institutional reforms aimed to strengthen the fight against drugs, (5) the signing of international agreements, and (6) acceptance of U.S. collaboration.[3] I have already mentioned the efforts made by the Mexican government in terms of the budget dedicated to fight drugs, seizures and eradication, arrests, and legal and institutional reforms. Let us see now how collaboration with the United States has been carried out.

During the Salinas administration, the U.S.-Mexico collaboration on the issue of drugs improved substantially, despite some minor friction. In 1992, for example, as a reaction to the U.S. Supreme Court decision authorizing kidnapping in foreign territory of persons prosecuted by American justice, the Mexican government implemented a bill aimed to regulate the "temporary stay of agents representing foreign governments offices that are in their country in charge of police, inspection or surveillance functions in law enforcement, as well as specialized technicians" (Government of Mexico 1992, 2). Also, as a way of protesting the U.S. Supreme Court decision, the Salinas government rejected, in 1992, the financial assistance channeled by Washington through the International Narcotics Control Program.

Nevertheless, in 1990, both countries launched the Northern Border Response Force, known in Spanish as Operación Halcón. Although this program was evaluated poorly in a General Accounting Office report, in May 1993, it was reported in the *1994 and 1995 International Narcotics Control Strategy Report*, released by the U.S. Department of State, as the "centerpiece" of U.S.-Mexican law enforcement cooperation and the

"focus of bilateral interdiction efforts." Its interest in collaborating with the United States moved the Mexican government to increase its involvement in antinarcotics operations in Central America and to collaborate with the Hemispheric System of Information. At the same time, the Salinas government improved radar surveillance in Mexican territory to detect planes carrying drugs, but there were some criticisms in the media alleging that this radar system had some blanks through which drug traffickers could penetrate into Mexico.

Zedillo took significant steps toward the creation of an alliance with the United States on the issue of drugs. In 1996, both governments established the High-Contact Level Group that was aimed to facilitate the exchange of information between the United States and Mexico and prevent a major diplomatic crisis. This collaboration produced joint operations, like the FBI investigation of the graves that were found in Ciudad Juarez on the U.S.-Mexican border at the end of 1999. In 1997, President Zedillo agreed to temporary extradition of drug traffickers to the United States. By May 2000, Mexico had extradited six Mexicans accused of drug trafficking, and there were another seven persons awaiting extradition, pending appeals court rulings. By May 2000, there were five Mexican citizens in the process of being extradited to the United States (White House 1998; Mexico, Attorney-General Offices 2000). We can expect more extradition cases in the future, especially after the Mexican Supreme Court ruled in January

2001 that the extradition of Mexicans to other countries is legal. Zedillo also accepted that U.S. ships and planes have access to Mexican airports and ports. There were also newspaper accounts of DEA agents' being allowed to carry guns in Mexican territory, but this has been denied officially by the Mexican government. It is also worth mentioning that the U.S. government is closely collaborating with the Mexican government in the training and selection of the members of the new Mexican antidrug unit created under Zedillo.

President Fox increased collaboration with the United States and has announced the creation of a Mexican Federal Agency of Investigations (a Mexican FBI), starting in December 2001, that will include an FBI training academy in Mexican territory. That clearly demonstrates a significant difference in the level of collaboration with the United States by the Mexican government compared to the past.

THE INEFFICIENT WAR

Despite all of the above-mentioned efforts, there are many weaknesses in the Mexican mechanisms to fight drugs. We can see this weakness in attempts to capture drug lords or corrupt officers. As has been mentioned, in January 1997, the Zedillo administration almost captured the Juarez Cartel leader Amado Carrillo, who escaped twenty minutes before the military arrived at his sister's wedding. In February 1997, one day before certification by the U.S. government was announced, Humberto Garcia Abrego, brother of the Gulf Cartel leader Juan Garcia Abrego, escaped from the Mexico City attorney general's headquarters without any logical explanation from the Mexican government. In this case, the Mexican government did not report this incident until the certification of Mexico was announced by U.S. Secretary of State Madeleine Albright. In June 1997, there was another scandal: four hundred kilos of seized cocaine disappeared from a local attorney general's office in Sonora along with the police who were in charge of the surveillance. In May 1999, Adan Amezcua, the methamphetamine czar, was released from prison because the judge ruled that the money laundering charges against him were not valid under the law at the time of the alleged offense. However, the most scandalous sign of institutional weakness was the escape from a maximum-security jail of Joaquin Chapo Guzman in January 2001. All these cases show how difficult the combat of drugs is in Mexico and the need to improve the performance of law enforcement institutions in Mexico.

POLICY OPTIONS

Given the institutional limitations that the Mexican government has in fighting drugs and the corrupting ability of the drug mafias, Mexico's options are limited. The first option is to do more of the same. This means combating drug trafficking with the same tools and with the same limitations as in the past. This option would imply the maintenance of the same levels of violence and corruption. In this sense, even when violence is not challenging Mexican governance, the threat coming from corruption could be more destabilizing. More of the same is supported by those who obtain benefits from the status quo: police officers and some Mexican politicians. The U.S. government supports this option only partially since it is conscious of the danger of having high degrees of corruption. Some of the supporters of this option are truly believers in the state's strength and think that drug traffickers can be treated like any other criminals and punished by the government. However, given the serious problems of corruption that the present strategy has not been able to solve, this policy option, without any modification, is difficult to support. But if this option is accompanied by a serious process of police and judicial reforms, it may receive more support if people perceive some degree of success. The problem is that these kinds of reforms take time to be implemented, and in the interim, the effects of corruption can be very damaging. At the same time, a question arises: if the Mexican state strengthens its offensive capabilities, it may provoke a reaction from the drug gangs that can transform drug-related violence into a real threat to governance in Mexico.

The second option is the Mexican state's declaring total war on drugs, without having the institutions capable of dealing with a virulent response of drug traffickers. This

option would work only if the Mexican government's pressure forced drug traffickers to move to other territories, as former attorney general Jorge Madrazo suggested in 1998. While this scenario is quite possible, and there is evidence that drug trafficking in the Caribbean has increased during recent years (Massing 2000), it is reasonable to expect higher levels of violence in Mexico if the option of total war is implemented. If we look at the volumes of drugs produced or transported through Mexico, the limited violence that drug trafficking generates in Mexico is quite surprising, compared to violence in other countries affected by the same phenomenon, such as Colombia. One possible explanation is that the Mexican state has purportedly maintained limited levels of confrontation with the drug gangs to maintain low levels of violence.[4]

A third option is to maintain the present antidrug strategy but do less. This option could be very attractive for a government that is in the midst of a political transition and needs high levels of stability. However, U.S. pressures could make this option difficult for the Fox administration, especially after the terrorist attacks in New York and Washington. In this context, it is quite reasonable to expect more pressures from Washington for security controls implemented by the Mexican government.

Finally, a fourth option is to modify in a radical way the present approach and, consequently, the present counterdrug strategy. That implies either the decriminalization of drug consumption or even the legalization of consumption, trafficking, and production of drugs. The option of decriminalization does not appear a good one for countries such as Mexico, which are still mainly producers or transit countries. Decriminalization would solve the problem of prosecuting millions of consumers in countries such as the United States, but it will not solve the challenges posed by drug traffickers in producer and transit countries. Legalization will clearly solve that problem, but it will probably aggravate the problem of consumption, which explains, in part, the United States' reluctance to talk about this possibility. The fact that the U.S. government is opposed to both legalization and decriminalization nullifies these options, in practical terms, for the next years.

At the present time, the most viable option is probably the first one: to maintain the present strategy of combating drugs while institutions are strengthened. If the process of institution building is successful, it is possible to think of the second option, a total war, as viable to force drug traffickers to move to other territories. Obviously, in this scenario, the solution of the problem for Mexico would mean a new problem for some other country.

CONCLUSIONS

Mexico's war on drugs has been determined by an international punitive regime constructed during many decades, U.S. pressures, the weakness of domestic law enforcement institutions, and the drug cartels' tremendous ability to corrupt. All these factors paint a very complex panorama for the Mexican government, with no margin for maneuver. Even though drugs do not represent a serious threat to Mexico in terms of domestic consumption or violence, the panorama gets darker when we talk about corruption. The possibility that corruption affects the ability of the Mexican state to guarantee the personal security of its citizens is very high. It is quite possible that drug-related corruption affects Mexico's ability to guarantee national and international security in a context of terrorist threats to the Western countries. In this perspective, it is feasible to expect strong U.S. pressures on the Mexican government to strengthen its ability to combat organized crime. This will probably lead to a closer collaboration between both countries in security matters that will make the U.S. government coresponsible for the failures and successes of the Mexican war on drugs. This collaboration will take place in the context of a rapid economic and cultural integration between both countries where there is little room for the historical anti-U.S. feelings. In the short run, it is difficult to expect big achievements in the combat of drugs. However, in the long run, if the process of institution building succeeds, drugs may become a health as well as a public security problem that does not challenge Mexico's governance. Meanwhile, the Mexican state has to deal with this problem in the best way it can.

Notes

1. The *Economist* mentioned the figure of $6 billion, quoting American drug czar Barry

McCaffrey (Drugs in the Americas 1997, 44). However, *Latin Trade* magazine said that according to U.S. and Mexican investigators, the profits of the drug trade laundered in Mexico are between $10 billion and $15 billion per year (Dirty laundry 1997).

2. In a press conference on 13 November 1997, Mexican Secretary of Foreign Affairs José Angel Gurría said that Mexico was spending around $1 billion per year (see Vargas 1997, 5).

3. These criteria are based on the arguments used by the U.S. government to grant certification every year.

4. Stanley Pimentel suggested that there have been arrangements between the state and drug traffickers that can explain the limited violence (see Pimentel 2000, 33-57).

References

Bailey, John, and Jorge Chabat. 2001. Public security and democratic governance: Challenges to Mexico and the United States. Report to Task Force. Center for Latin American Studies, Edmund A. Walsh School of Foreign Service, Georgetown University, Washington, DC. Mimeographed.

Chabat, Jorge. 1994. Drug trafficking in the U.S.-Mexican relations: What you see is what you get. In *Drug trafficking in the Americas*, edited by Bruce M. Bagley and William O. Walker III. New Brunswick, NJ: Transaction Publishing/North-South Center.

Constantine, Thomas A. 1996. Statement before the House Appropriations Committee Subcommittee on Commerce, Justice, State, the Judiciary, and Related Agencies regarding fiscal year 1997 appropriations. May 1. Retrieved from www.usdoj.gov/dea/pubs/cngrtest/ct960501.htm.

Dirty laundry. 1997. *Latin Trade*. September.

Drug Strategies. 1994. A review of US international drug control policy. Mimeographed.

Drugs in the Americas: Time for retreat? 1997. *Economist*, 8 March, 44.

Government of Mexico. 1992. *Diario Oficial de la Federación*. Mexico, D.F.: Secretaría de Gobernacion, CDLXVI(3):2. 3 July.

Lupsha, Peter A. 1995. Transnational narco-corruption and narco investment: A focus on Mexico. *Transnational Organized Crime* 1(1, spring).

Massing, Michael. 2000. The narco-state? *New York Review of Books*, 15 June, 24-29.

Mexico, Attorney-General Office. 2000. La lucha de México contra el Narcotráfico (Reduccón de la Oferta). Mimeographed.

Mexico, Secretaria de Salud. 1999. El consumo de drogas en México. Mexico, D.F.: Secretaria de Salud.

Pimentel, Stanley. 2000. The nexus of organized crime and politics in Mexico. In *Organized crime and democratic governability: Mexico and the U.S.-Mexican borderlands*, edited by John Bailey and Roy Godson, 33-57. Pittsburgh, PA: University of Pittsburgh Press.

Reuter, Peter, and David Ronfeldt. 1992, Quest for integrity: The Mexican-US drug issue in the 1980s. *Journal of Interamerican Studies and World Affairs* 34 (3): 89-153.

U.S. Department of Justice, Drug Enforcement Administration. 2002. Today's major drug trafficking organizations in Mexico. Retrieved from http://www.usdoj.gov/dea/traffickers/mexico.htm.

U.S. State Department. 1994. *International narcotics control strategy report*. Washington, D.C.: Department of State Publication 10145.

U.S. State Department. 1995. *International narcotics control strategy report*. Washington, D.C.: Department of State Publication 10246.

U.S. State Department. 2000. *International narcotics control strategy report*. Retrieved from www.state.gov/g/inl/rls/nrcpt/2000.

————. 2001. *International narcotics control strategy report 2000*. Retrieved from www.state.gov/g/inl/rls/nrcrpt/2001.

Vargas, Rosa Elvira. 1997. Esencialmente trasnacional, el tráfico ilegal de armas: Gaviria. *La Jornada*, 14 November, 5.

Walker, William O., III. 1981. *Drug control in the Americas*. Albuquerque: University of New Mexico Press.

White House. 1998. U.S.-Mexico counterdrug cooperation. Mimeographed.

The Drug Market in Iran

By FARIBORZ RAISDANA

with the cooperation of AHMAD GHARAVI NAKHJAVANI

ABSTRACT: This article reviews the history of the opium and heroin market in Iran, presents recent figures on the economics of drug trafficking, summarizes factors that influence supply and demand, and quantitatively analyzes the market. It analyzes economic causes and motives of supply and demand, plus risk of seizure, and the socioeconomic characteristics of consumers and retailers. All these factors support conclusions about price trends, their causes and results, the function of the market and the individual motives of its people of the different socioeconomic groups, particularly the youth.

Fariborz Raisdana was born in Tehran and educated in Tehran (National University of Iran) and London (London School of Economics and City University). He taught at the National University of Iran, Tehran University, and now is a researcher at the University of Social Welfare and Rehabilitation. He has published fourteen books on development, urban and regional planning, the economy of Iran, money and inflation, social pathology, poverty and discrimination, and political economy.

Ahmad Gharavi Nakhjavani was born in Tehran and graduated from Azad Tehran University in economics. He has been the educator of management in the faculty of Azad University, Tehran, since 1998. He has cooperated with Iranian bulletins and has published articles on poverty, development, stagflation, and the drug market in Iran.

I N Iranian culture, the reciprocal emotional relationship between parents and children is still strong and long lasting. Consequently, the drug addiction of Iranian youth have caused families to press the government to control drugs and combat drug traffickers (Mahyar and Jazayer 1998; Dezhkam 2000). For its part, the government is inclined to control drugs because the formal political Shiite ideology (according to interpretation of the majority of clergy) views the prevalence of drugs as a conspiracy of the enemy to weaken the *Ommat* (Muslim people of our country) (Iran in the front line of drug battle 1999). Therefore, the huge annual human losses and economic damages of drug consumption and trafficking have caused the government to give priority to controlling the drug supply. In my opinion, the government is also obliged to sympathize with and take responsibility for drug control as a way of alleviating the negative attitude the governments of Western countries have toward human rights in Iran.

OPIUM AND HEROIN
ADDICTION IN IRAN

Historical background

Opiates and hashish are derived from plants indigenous to Iran. Historical evidence and documents clearly show that Iranian people have known psychotropic, medical, and nutritional qualities of these plants for thousands of years. For example, Herodotus (fifth century B.C.) refers to this in his writings. The writings of both Rhazes and Avicenna (tenth and eleventh centuries) refer to the sedative and tranquilizing effect of opiates.

The kings of the Safavid dynasty, who ruled for almost 200 years beginning at the latter part of the fifteenth century, established central authority, expanded Iran's territory, and promoted economic growth and commerce. During this period, abuse of opium surged. To control it, Abbas II, the most important and powerful king of this period, combined the use of force with Shiite Islamic ideology. Despite the help of scholars steeped in the scientific methods of their time, this effort marked the first failure of state intervention against drug abuse and addiction. About 130 years after the Safavid dynasty, during the Qajar dynasty, the use of opium increased. At that time, opium was usually taken by mouth and rarely smoked. Also during this period, lower-class rural, tribal, and urban people began using opium.

During the eighteenth and the first half of the nineteenth century, opium was cultivated in Iran mostly for domestic consumption. But this changed in the second half of the nineteenth century when the commercial potential of this substance increased substantially with the sudden emergence of opium use in Europe and poppy cultivation in China. At that time, use of opium in Iran and Europe was socially acceptable. In fact, Iran managed, albeit with much effort, to obtain England's permission to export opium to India (Mavvad-e Mokhader 2000).

National leaders were motivated to wage a political, social, and ideological campaign against opium abuse because of a combination of circumstances. These included the constitutional movement (1908), and the social democratic movements before and after that, which replaced the old despotic monarchy regime with a new parliamentary system; the development of democracy; participation of the urban middle class in political and public affairs; and new ideas of social democracy and social justice. Consequently, the first legislation to control opium use was enacted in 1911. This law phased in the prohibition of nonpharmaceutical use of opium during a period of eight years. The government issued and distributed ration coupons to opium addicts. By 1926, nearly 8 percent of the government revenue came from levies on opium. But the passage of the 1911 law failed to decrease the use of opium, and contrary to all expectations, exports increased. In 1922, the government had no choice but to ban importation of narcotic substances (Mavvad-e Mokhader 2000).

Pursuant to international pressure in 1928, during the reign of Pahlavi I, another law was passed, giving the opium monopoly to the government. Meanwhile, the government also committed itself to gradually reducing poppy cultivation and demand, as well as providing treatment facilities. Only pharmacies were permitted to sell opium. Nevertheless, within ten years, the land under poppy cultivation increased 1.5-fold, and opium export jumped from 291.5 tons in 1928 to 448.3 tons in 1938. Whereas the land under cultivation increased by 4.4 percent per year during this ten-year period, the

population had increased by only around 1.5 percent in the first decades of twentieth century (Mavvad-e Mokhader 2000).

After the fall of Pahlavi I in 1941 and World War II, an open political climate developed. The nationalist government of Mohammed Mossadegh (1950-1953) did much to promote democracy and social justice and to protect national interests. It forced the British government to accept Iran's demand for nationalization of its oil industry, but Mossadegh's government was overthrown by a Central Intelligence Agency–aided coup d'etat. During Mossadegh's government, a special commission had been established to plan for the prohibition of poppy cultivation, to establish drug treatment facilities, and to make some trade illicit. The Alcoholics and Opium Abusers Anonymous Society was also established.

At the grassroots level, the political democratic movement effectively reined in opium abuse. Nevertheless, in 1943, an astonishing 1.5 million people of the total population of 14 million were estimated to have used opium. In 1949, the United Nations convened a special conference, which proposed a quota system for global opium cultivation: 50 percent for Turkey and 15 percent for Iran.

Finally in 1955, the Iranian parliament passed one of the most important laws relating to consumption and production of opium—by banning poppy cultivation and opium use entirely. After the 1953 coup d'etat, the artificial prosperity of the middle urban classes, especially in Tehran, along with waves of migration to the cities, widened the gap among social classes. Meanwhile, poverty and unemployment caused by opium use continued to increase. Heroin and morphine use among wealthier families, including the Shah's, became prevalent. After 1955, law enforcement applied stricter measures, and officers received bonuses for seizing narcotics. Nevertheless, consumption surged—especially in such cities as Hamadan, Kerman, Mashhad, Zabol, and Tehran—as a result of social contradictions, disposable income of the upper classes, poverty, discrimination against the lower classes, and possibly the illicit cultivation, importation, and production of heroin. In 1959, for example, 5,225 kilograms of opium and 4,500 kilograms of heroin were seized. In 1965, 13,117 kilograms and 17,200 kilograms were seized, respectively. In 1968, Iran set the world record in narcotics seizures, as it has continued to do (Mavvad-e Mokhader 2000).

Continuation of poppy cultivation in Pakistan and Turkey and the inability to control cultivation in the southern and western parts of the country prompted Iran in 1968 to again permit the cultivation of poppy in special government-controlled areas. For opium addicts age fifty years and older, opium ration coupons were issued, but military courts meted out severe punishments, including death sentences, to drug traffickers. Between 1969 and 1977, forty to fifty death sentences were reported. The dual policy of strict control of supply and relatively liberal regulation of consumption

continued until 1979. This policy failed to produce the desired results, both socially and economically.

In mid-1975, nearly 170,000 addicts were registered, and an estimated 200,000 to 500,000 were not. At that time, 180 tons of opium equivalent was being consumed. Estimates in 1976, based on urine test sampling in big cities, indicated that nearly 2.5 percent of the population was addicted, that is, nearly 400,000 of the 15 million urban population. However, more precise studies indicate that this number is a significant underestimation. In my opinion, the total number of serious drug addicts (excluding accidental and recreational use) was not less than 1 million people; therefore, the total consumption of opiate substances was at least 350 tons (Mavvad-e Mokhader 2000).

Improvement of economic conditions in Iran after 1973 led to the establishment of a number of rehabilitation centers, but they were not effective in reducing the number of substance users.

After the Islamic revolution

After the victory of the Islamic revolution in 1979, despite the drug addiction of some of the new managers and some members of the clergy, the new revolutionary leaders and judges of revolutionary courts strove to counteract the effects of drug abuse. The managers of the Islamic revolution put the blame squarely on the conspiracies of the "Great Satan," the West, and counterrevolutionaries. They tried to stamp out drug abuse by suppression, arrest, execution, and imprisonment of addicts and sellers of narcotics. Ayatollah Sadegh Khalkhali, a religious judge, was given the responsibility of arresting and executing a large number—probably thousands—of addicts and sellers of opiate substances. He also tried and executed many ministers, parliamentarians, and officials of the former regime, which put him in the international spotlight. All drug rehabilitation hospitals were closed. Especially after the start of the Iran-Iraq war, keeping a drug addict in a hospital, even a private hospital, warranted punishment of hospital managers, such as demotion and even dismissal. Instead, special camps were established for addicts, who were sent to them in groups as prisoners.

In 1983, special rehabilitation centers were established under the supervision of the State Welfare Organization. They received only addicts whom the courts referred to them. Quarters were overcrowded and conditions squalid.

Until 1987 and the end of the Iran-Iraq war, all efforts focused on reduction of supply. In many cases, the addicts and small addict/pushers were dealt with in the same way as traffickers. From 1974 to 1988, according to published numbers, 310 tons of narcotics were seized, of which 10 percent was heroin. In 1988, a strict policy was reestablished, and the State Expediency Council, which lacks legislative power and can give only advisory opinions in times of crisis, enacted a new law. It enacted more severe punishments so that mere consumption of a drug became a punishable offence. The Drug Control Headquarters (DCH) was placed under the direct supervision of the president, as it remained in 2001 (*Proceedings and papers* 1999; Doran-e Emrooz 2001).

The minister of health and the president of Islamic Republic of Iran Broadcasting became members of the DCH. Assets confiscated from traffickers became the property of the DCH to finance its planning and research operations. Since the establishment of the DCH, 250 officers have been killed, and more have been injured in their fight against the illicit trade in narcotics. In some years, as many as 500 traffickers were executed; sometimes a body would be left hanging on the gallows for many days. On many occasions, police raided areas that addicts and drug retailers frequented and sometimes razed large settlements to the ground, transferring the inhabitants elsewhere, only to have drug dealers simply shift to another location, spreading this disease as they went.

Despite all these activities, drug addiction continues to increase. Diminishing consumption has been reported during the past ten to thirteen years, but this is simply due to the fact that more and more users eat opiate substances instead of smoking them (Chearlo 1999). Eating opium is more economical (despite its somewhat different effect) because it is a more efficient way of achieving ecstasy (*Proceedings and papers* 1999).

The eastern borders of the country continue to be the main points of entry and narcotics trafficking. For the big traffickers and small retailers who face unemployment, poverty, and addiction, supplying narcotics, despite its risks, is an economically viable proposition.

Meanwhile, signs of popular fatigue from this costly and futile campaign are appearing. Some officials and writers have begun voicing the need for more liberalization. Some call for more international assistance in the eastern areas of the country. Other critics believe that the West is not really interested in stopping supply, consumption, and transit. They argue that some amount of narcotics is necessary to calm conflict-ridden and aggressive social conditions in the West, especially for the unruly youth. They also argue that eliminating opiate substances paves the way for production of more harmful synthetic drugs that are much harder to control.

There are also those who believe that in the absence of sincere and honest cooperation from the global community, Iran should be allowed to open controlled corridors for the passage of narcotic substances (*Political declaration guiding principles* 1999). This, they believe, would allow Iran to control spilling and leakage, while Iran could also use some of this narcotic for supervised distribution to its duly registered addicts. This way, the country would not have to bear the heavy burden of fighting traffickers mainly for the interest of Western countries. Those who advocate establishing a global fund to finance alternative crops in Afghanistan face the same Western clandestine policy of wanting to have some opiate substances coming into Europe. Faced with this situation, they resort to innovative and radical approaches or opt for a laissez-faire policy.

OPIUM AND ITS DERIVATIVES

This article focuses on narcotic opium derivatives, which constitute the principal narcotics being imported, consumed, and trafficked in Iran. At least five types of poppy products are consumed in Iran (Chearlo 1999; *Community drug profile #1* 1999; *Community drug profile #2* 1999; *Community drug profile #3* 2000).

Opium. The most commonly known opiate is derived from seedpods of the fruit of the opium poppy plant (called Khashkhash in Iran) by incising the fruit and collecting the sap. Farmers incise the outer skin of the fruit, and after ten to twelve hours, a sticky brown sap appears from the egg-shaped bulb (the size of a pigeon egg to that of a chicken egg). When the extracted sap is rubbed on a smooth surface, its color changes from milky white to brown. The more the extracted sap is rubbed, the more moisture evaporates and the drier the opium becomes. The final product is rolled in ten- to fifteen-centimeter rolls and tablets (½ gram) or cakes (30 to 40 grams). This type of opium is usually dry or semidry.

Crude opium. Boiling the bulb of the opium poppy thickens it and produces crude opium. The product, which contains less morphine than opium does, is usually packed in cakes or in bulk forms.

Morphine and heroin. Morphine, or monoacetylmorphine, is the most active ingredient of opium. Opium contains about 10 percent morphine. Heroin, or diacetylmorphine, is made by combining morphine and anhydric acid. This is the most harmful opiate, and its smoke is inhaled or injected intravenously. Heroin, depending on its purity, is four to ten times more potent than opium.[1]

Shiray. Another derivative of opium, shiray is probably used exclusively in Iran. When opium is smoked in a *Vafour*, or the opium-smoker's pipe, the residue left inside its vase-shaped head is scraped off and boiled in water. After a number of boilings, the remaining juice is heated to thicken it, producing a thick, black or dark brown substance. This is called shiray. Shiray is smoked by means of an instrument called a *Negari*.

PRICES

Trends

The price of narcotic substances has increased in Iran along with general inflation. However, inflation-adjusted prices have fallen substantially. From 1990 to 1996, the rate of price escalation for consumer goods has been much higher than the price increase for opium. Only in two years, 1997 and 1998, did the price of opium in Tehran increase sharply, but it came down again in 1999. It is notable that during the period from 1992 to 1994, the nominal price of opium declined. The real price of Tehran opium from 1990 to 2001 (see Figure 1) declined by two-thirds

between 1990 and 1999 (Mavvad-e Mokhader 2000; Survey on drugs in Iran 2000a, 2000b; Masraf-e Mavvad-e Mokhader Dar Iran 2000; Ghachagh-e Mavvad-e Makhader 2000).

Counteractivities on the borders and around Tehran and a simultaneous U.K. mission in Iran in March 2000 increased the price in 2001, but the price could not be sustained and again decreased from June to September of 2001, the most recent data available. Opium and other opiates in Iran have become cheaper, and many users can better afford to pay for narcotics. This is not true, however, for hard-core heroin addicts and the unemployed, whose income has fallen, and they must resort to theft and other offences to meet their addiction needs.

A number of factors influence prices of narcotics in Tehran, including production in Afghanistan, arrest of traffickers, and seizure of narcotics shipments. A regression of the price is presented against the previous year's production in Afghanistan. More than 75 percent of the change in the price of opium in Tehran can be explained by changes in previous years in the harvest of the poppy crop and opium production. Figure 2 shows the relationship between the decline in the real price of opium in Tehran and the previous year's production. Although the mere existence of a relationship is not proof of causality, it can be concluded that the main reason behind the decline in the real price of opium was probably the increase in production and prevalence of trafficking. A number of studies and various calculated

FIGURE 1
AVERAGE REAL PRICE OF OPIUM IN TEHRAN FROM 1990 TO 2000, IN 1990 RIALS

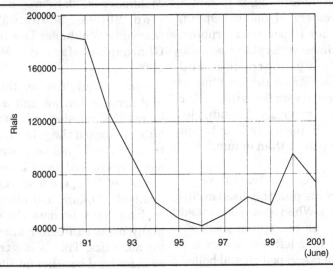

SOURCE: Mavvad-e Mokhader 2000; Survey on drug in Iran 2000a, 2000b; Masraf-e Mavvad-e Mokhader Dar Iran 2000; Ghachagh-e Mavvad-e Makhader 2000; data collection by researcher.

statistical coefficients indicate that the campaign and interdiction activities against illicit narcotics trade has played no significant role in changing the real price of opium and its derivatives (*Global illicit drug trends 2000* 2000; *World drug report* 1997; *Annual opium poppy survey 2000* 2000).

Value added by stage of distribution

Narcotics prices differ by region; namely, they increase with distance from the eastern borders (see Table 1). Naturally, as the price of narcotic drugs increases, there will also be an added value as a result of shifting of shipments. The variation in prices in twenty-six regions and provinces in 1998 suggests that the principal factor is distance from point of entry. Zahedan, the closest city to the eastern border with Afghanistan, was selected for this review of prices for narcotic substances. Figure 3 illustrates this close relationship. Estimated regression equations show that every 100 kilometers adds 145,000 rials to the price of opium, approximately 8 percent of the base price in Zahedan. Since the point of entry of narcotics cannot be Sistan and Baluchistan Province for all regions of the country, Khorasan Province was also included.

Controlling for distance, the average price of opium that entered the country from Khorasan was about 770,000 rials higher than the price of opium that entered from Sistan and Baluchistan.

FIGURE 2
**THE RELATIONSHIP BETWEEN THE REAL PRICE OF OPIUM
IN TEHRAN AND OPIUM PRODUCTION IN AFGHANISTAN**

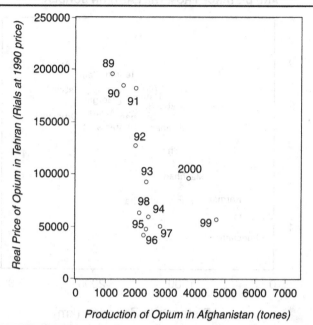

Production of Opium in Afghanistan (tones)

SOURCE: *Global illicit drug trends 2000* 2000; *World drug report* 1997; *Annual opium poppy survey 2000* 2000; data collection by researcher.

TABLE 1
**DIRECT COSTS FOR THE CAMPAIGN AGAINST NARCOTICS
TRAFFICKING AND ADDICTION (AT 3,500 RIALS TO THE DOLLAR)**

Expenses	Cost (U.S.$)
Constructing watch posts and guard houses, stringing barbed wire, excavating canals, patrolling border roads, deploying armed forces	173,067,000
Wages and salaries, rations, clothing, accommodations, and so forth	
Depreciation and loss of vehicles, armaments, helicopters, and communications facilities	
Payments to the families of officers injured or killed (120 killed and 500 disabled in 1998) and monthly allowance to 3,000 families of killed or injured officers	
Medical, rehabilitation, and detention expenditure for addicts; 18,000 rehabilitation cases	110,234,000
Costs for 30,000 outpatients, 200,000 arrests, 250,000 court cases, and detention of 100,000 drug-related prisoners	
Prevention expenditures relating to traffickers, substance abuse (educational, cultural advertising), television programs, ministry of education	32,905,000
Total direct costs	316,206,000

SOURCE: Drug Control Headquarters (1998).

FIGURE 3
**THE RELATIONSHIP BETWEEN OPIUM PRICE
AND DISTANCE FROM THE EASTERN BORDER**

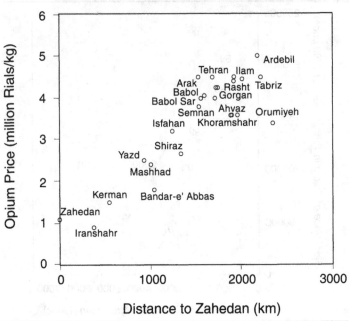

DISTRIBUTION

Surveys and studies show that narcotics use is prevalent (Mavvad-e Mokhader 2000; Survey on drugs in Iran 2000a, 2000b; Masraf-e Mavvad-e Mokhader Dar Iran 2000; Ghachagh-e Mavvad-e Makhader 2000). Between 1993 and 1998, narcotics seizures increased twofold, while the number of people arrested for drug trafficking increased fivefold. Researchers believe that the increase in seizures was mostly due to increased opium production in Afghanistan, not changes in efficiency or method of seizures, interdictions, and arrests. In other words, although narcotics transit has increased, per capita seizures for each trafficker have declined

substantially, from 5.5 kilograms in 1992 to less than 2 kilograms in 1998. Drug traffickers constitute an increasing share of the total prison population, rising from 26 percent in 1992 to 42 percent in 1998 (Mavvad-e Mokhader 2000; Survey on drugs in Iran 2000a, 2000b; Masraf-e Mavvad-e Mokhader Dar Iran 2000; Ghachagh-e Mavvad-e Makhader 2000).

The number of persons engaged in distribution of narcotics appears to have increased greatly. Probably the main reasons for this phenomenon are the increase in transit of narcotics, the higher level of domestic consumption, and the economic recession and consequent unemployment from 1992 to 1998.

TABLE 2
NUMBER OF REFERRALS TO REHABILITATION CENTERS,
BY FREQUENCY OF REFERRALS

| Year | Past Record of Quitting | | | | | Total |
	None	Once	Twice	Three times	More than three times	
1998						
n	10,959	9,253	5,161	2,848	2,462	30,683
%	35.7	30.1	17	9.2	8	100
1999						
n	12,215	10,566	6,171	3,770	3,838	34,560
%	33.4	29	16.8	10.3	10.5	100
Annual growth rate (1998-1999) (%)	11	14	20	32	56	19

SOURCE: Drug Control Headquarters (1998).

DRUG CONTROL

As for the performance of drug enforcement agencies in terms of quantities seized and traffickers arrested, the main reason for the increase is the higher production of opium in Afghanistan (*World drug report* 1997; *Annual opium poppy survey 2000* 2000). In fact, the relationship between seizures in Iran and production in Afghanistan is almost linear; the correlation coefficient is close to 85 percent. The principal source of fluctuation in quantities seized is not the efficiency of narcotics enforcement agencies but the efficiency of production and transit of narcotics through Iran. No meaningful relationship was found between narcotics seizures and a number of other factors, including costs incurred. Direct costs to government agencies are shown in Table 1: in 1998, more than U.S.$316 million was spent on the campaign against narcotic drugs (DCH 1998).

Table 2 shows number of referrals to rehabilitation or treatment cen-

ters in 1998 and 1999, distinguishing among patients by frequency of prior referral.

Only 33 percent of referrals to rehabilitation centers in 1999 were for first timers. Although 67 percent had a past record of referral, that percentage does not necessarily comprise all those whose treatment was unsuccessful. Table 2 also shows that as frequency of referral increases, so does annual growth rate.

CONSUMPTION OF
NARCOTIC DRUGS

Estimating consumption

The DCH and other relevant organizations, as well as most experts, estimate the number of hard-core addicts at 1.15 million and recreational users (light addicts) at another 880,000. In addition, according to the Rehabilitation Center of Iran and the University of Social Welfare, 1 million to 4 million Iranians are occasional users. Light users' total consumption of opium is nearly

TABLE 3

NUMBER OF ADDICTS AND AMOUNT OF NARCOTICS CONSUMED, 1997 TO 1999

| | Narcotic | | | |
User	Opium (shiray and opium)	Shiray (opium residue)	Heroin and Morphine	Total (kilograms)
Hard-core addicts				
1997-1999 (kg)	800,000	100,000	250,000	1,150,000
Daily average (g/day)	2.5	0.65	0.3	
Light addicts (recreational use and more daily average)				
1997-1999 (kg)	600,000	50,000	100,000	750,000
Daily average (g/day)	0.35	0.1	0.05	
Light addicts (recreational and random use)				
1997-1999 (kg)	100,000	20,000	10,000	130,000
Daily average (g/day)	0.15	0.05	0.01	
Total				
1997-1999 (kg)	1,500,000	170,000	360,000	2,030,000
Daily average (g/day)	1.5	0.42	0.22	

fifty metric tons per year. However, many experts believe that the population of hard-core and light addicts is between 2.5 million and 2.6 million because approximately 500,000 addicts are unknown or clandestine. Mostly, these people are opium addicts (oral form), and their per capita consumption is not very high. On the basis of sampling and review of referrals to rehabilitation centers, I estimate that the number of addicts in Iran is close to the numbers stated above. The exaggerated figures of unofficial sources have no sound basis and do not correspond to production levels in Afghanistan. Also, underestimates are given out for propaganda or other political reasons.

Using the prevalence figures in Table 3, the annual consumption per capita in Iran can be estimated (see Table 4).

TABLE 4

ANNUAL CONSUMPTION OF DRUGS IN IRAN (PURE OPIUM EQUIVALENT)

Narcotic	Total Tons
Opium and shiray	528
Heroin and morphine	58.4

Estimation of the amount of heroin and morphine consumed in 1999 in Iran is the equivalent of 586.4 tons of opium. Table 5 shows the quantity of opium produced in Southwest Asia and distributed in 1999. In Afghanistan and Pakistan, 4,574 tons were produced; regional consumption in Iran, Pakistan, and Afghanistan was 1,481 tons of opium equivalent (17.4 percent opium and 15 percent heroin). Deducting quantities seized, the net export of the region is estimated at 1,748 tons (including real export and quantity stored for export).

TABLE 5

**DISTRIBUTION OF OPIUM PRODUCED
IN SOUTHWEST ASIA (1999 ESTIMATES)**

Number	Narcotic	Percentage	Quantity (metric tons)
1	Production of opium in Afghanistan and Pakistan[a]	100	4,574
2	Domestic consumption in Iran		528[b]
3	Domestic consumption in Pakistan and Afghanistan[c]	17.4	270
			(conservative estimate)
4	Domestic consumption of heroin in Iran (opium equivalent)		58[d]
5	Domestic consumption of heroin in Pakistan and Afghanistan (opium equivalent)	15	625
6	Total consumption in the region	32.4	1,481
7	Excess in the region (no. 1 – no. 6 = no.7)	67.6	3,093
8	Seizure in Iran (opium equivalent)	9.7	445
9	Seizure in Pakistan (opium equivalent)	13.1	600 (estimated)
10	Total seizure in the region (no. 8 + no. 9 = no. 10)	23	1,045
11	Export (no. 7 – no. 10 = no. 11)	44.8	2,048
12	Seized outside of the region	6	300 (estimated)
13	Net export (no. 11 – no. 12 = no. 13)	38	1,748
14	Net export through Iran, assuming 80 percent leaves the country	35.8	1,638
15	Total possible consumption of heroin	53	1,748 + 58 + 625 = 2,431

a. Of this amount, 9 tons relate to Pakistan, and the remainder to Afghanistan.

b. Assuming an average purity of 65 percent for opium in Iran, 528 tons of pure opium would be adequate for 812 tons of consumption.

c. Close to 90 percent relates to Pakistan.

d. Assuming an average purity of 20 percent for heroin in Iran, 5.84 tons of pure heroin would be adequate for 29.2 tons of consumption. As in previous calculations, opium equivalent would be 10 × 5.8 = 58 tons.

Stored narcotics for domestic use have a useful life of less than one year and are therefore not included in these calculations (Mahyar and Jazayer 1998; Dezhkam 2000; *Drugs, money and laundering* 1998; *Annual report on the state of the drugs problem in the European Union* 2000; *Annual opium poppy survey* 2000; *Community drug profile #1* 1999; *Community drug profile #2* 1999; *Community drug profile #3* 2000).

Tehran prices

Consumer prices for different narcotic substances (with average purity) in Tehran in October 2000 are presented in Table 6. Narcotics prices are compared with average prices for food and nonfood items in Table 7.

In Tehran, one gram of heroin costs the same as one kilogram of red meat, three kilograms of average-quality rice, and more than ten kilograms of potatoes or two books. Or

TABLE 6
RETAIL STREET PRICES
OF NARCOTICS IN TEHRAN

Narcotic	Minimum Retail Price (rial/gram)	Maximum Retail Price (rial/gram)
Opium	5,300	7,500
Heroin	20,000	24,000
Shiray of opium residue	7,500	13,000
Morphine	13,200	15,000

SOURCE: Direct inquiry in different parts of Tehran.

TABLE 7
AVERAGE PRICES OF
SELECTED ITEMS IN TEHRAN

Description	Average Price (in rials)
Kilogram of red meat	22,000
Kilogram of rice	3,000-12,000
Kilogram of potatoes	2,000
One hundred grams of instant coffee	35,000
Bottle of smuggled whiskey	170,000
Bottle of home-brewed vodka on the black market	10,000
Man's suit	500,000
Woman's overcoat	200,000
Two-hundred–page book	10,000

the price of one gram of opium equals the cost of three hundred to four hundred grams of red meat.

Since addicts consume different quantities, depending on the type of narcotic they use, it is better to compare their monthly expenditure for narcotics with items listed above. Surveys show that the red meat equivalent in a month to support their habit costs heroin addicts five kilograms, an opium addict twenty kilograms, and a shiray addict ten kilograms.

TABLE 8
ABSOLUTE AND RELATIVE SEX
PREVALENCE OF REFERRALS TO THE
RECEPTION, TREATMENT, AND FOLLOW-
UP UNIT OF ADDICTS IN IRAN AND
TEHRAN PROVINCE, 1999

Sex	Tehran Province		Iran	
	n	%	n	%
Men	7,275	97	21,835	97
Women	260	3	675	3
Total	7,535	100	22,510	100

SOURCE: State Welfare Organization (1998, 1999).

CONSUMERS

Sex

Of those who self-referred to a treatment center in Iran, women accounted for 3 percent, both throughout Iran and in Tehran (see Table 8), but the real number seems to be higher because the status of women in the family and deprivation of women would result in few referrals. Regardless, the number of women addicts is increasing, and many surveys indicate that more and more women are using narcotics. It is also reported that women who are at risk of physical and sexual abuse are four times more likely to abuse narcotics (State Welfare Organization of Islamic Republic of Iran 1998, 1999).

Education

More than 74 percent of those who came to self-referral centers in 1998

TABLE 9

RELATIVE AND ABSOLUTE PREVALENCE OF EDUCATIONAL LEVEL OF REFERRALS TO RECEPTION, TREATMENT, AND FOLLOW-UP UNIT FOR ADDICTS IN TEHRAN PROVINCE, 1995

Education	n	%
Illiterate	446	5.9
Elementary	2,188	29.1
Ninth grade	2,932	38.9
Secondary	1,497	19.8
Junior college	242	3.2
University degree	179	2.4
Postgraduate	51	0.7
Total	7,535	100

SOURCE: State Welfare Organization (1998, 1999).

were illiterate or had less than a secondary-level education, whereas only 3 percent of referrals had a university education (see Table 9). If those who came to self-referral centers of their own volition were better educated, then it could be concluded that level of education of addicts was lower than this statistical sample's.

Income

Approximately 36.1 percent of self-referrals to treatment centers in 1998 earned less per month than 200,000 rials; 23.5 percent between 200,000 and 300,000 rials; 20.9 percent between 300,000 and 600,000 rials; 7.6 percent between 600,000 and 800,000 rials; and 12 percent more than 800,000 rials. Thus, more than 80 percent who went to self-referral centers earned less than 600,000 rials per month. The monthly weighted income of referrals was calculated to be 389,000 rials. Considering that 70 percent of

referrals were married and had an average of two children, and that the minimum wage in that year was 400,000 rials, the majority of addicts can hardly afford the bare necessities of life, even without the expense of narcotics. (The average monthly income of addicts in Tehran is higher than that throughout Iran.)

Narcotics-related expenditures

Weighted average monthly expenses for narcotics at rehabilitation centers in 1998 was close to 399,000 rials (93,230 rials per week). In other words, monthly expenditures on narcotics by this group were more than their monthly income.

This group could not pay for their living expenses let alone pay for the cost of their addiction. That is one of the reasons addicts sell narcotics to earn money and why there is a close relationship between addiction and crime.

Employment status of addicts

Employment status of addicts who entered rehabilitation centers in 1998 is shown in Figure 4. Although this chart divides numbers of addicts into various occupations, it is useless without comparable data from the general population. Referrals to the rehabilitation centers are mostly in their productive years; therefore, comparison of the ratio of addicts with the ratio of people of productive age throughout the total workforce would give better results. The official unemployment rate in 1998 was about 14 percent, whereas unemployment among addicts was 24 percent, which indicates a probable

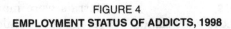

FIGURE 4
EMPLOYMENT STATUS OF ADDICTS, 1998

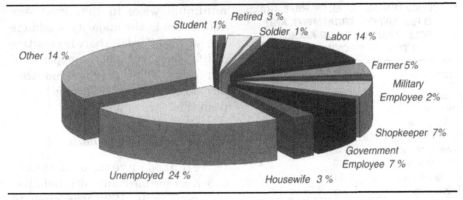

Retired 3 %
Student 1%
Soldier 1%
Labor 14 %
Other 14 %
Farmer 5%
Military
Employee 2%
Shopkeeper 7%
Government
Employee 7 %
Unemployed 24 %
Housewife 3 %

meaningful relationship between unemployment and addiction. On the other hand, the 7 percent of addicts who were government employees may seem high, but in the total gainfully employed population, the ratio of government employees was 12 percent.

SUMMARY AND CONCLUSION

From the foregoing, eight conclusions become clear:

1. Consumption of narcotics (i.e., demand) in Iran is mainly influenced by fundamental factors of unemployment and poverty, social problems such as discrimination, extraordinary and easy money making of the minority rich on one hand, and the absence of social amenities and leisure for the majority of the people on the other. In fact, many entertainments, pleasures, and social and private freedoms, which many people find necessary and normal, are prohibited. For this reason, young people

are usually the easiest prey for narcotics dealers.

2. Despite the fact that the real price of opium and heroin have decreased, the profitability of supply is still high. The reasons are that the total trafficking and total demand have increased, while poverty and unemployment are still widespread, particularly in eastern regions. A quarter of the drug addicts are themselves small-scale retailers because of increasing unemployment and income deficiencies of a huge part of society. But these distributors in turn are determinant factors of continued supply.

3. Among noneconomic factors influencing demand, there are cultural and social conflicts as well as privation, discrimination, civil degradation, and political pressure.

4. Noneconomic factors influencing supply include pressure from the former reactionary, despotic, and suppressive government in Afghanistan; absence of efficient, systemic strategy and management for control of demand and supply in both Iran

and Pakistan; lack of effective, stable, and believable officials; lack of direct international cooperation; prevalent corruption; and absence of fair and humanitarian policies for Afghani immigrants (which, in Iran, despite all assistance, is mainly due to lack of financial resources and recently to internal economic crisis).

5. Drug demand reduction efforts might best be directed toward a campaign against unemployment, poverty, and injustice. Also needed are improvements in social conditions, particularly for the youth, as well as political development and democracy. In fact, more freedom, entertainment, sports facilities, recreation, and a generally happy life are also vital for the DCH in Iran.

6. Strict enforcement, instead of more humanitarian policies, is counterproductive; that is, many addicts are victims of socioeconomic disorder, but even young people, considered criminals, become supply factors.

7. As long as demand continues to increase and supply is profitable, the transit of opium and heroin from Iran to Europe will continue. The total amount of consumption of drugs in Iran may fluctuate, but regardless, a considerable share of the production in Afghanistan may pass to European destinations by way of Iran.

8. Price increases can motivate cultivation, trafficking, and retailing and can violate risk-to-profit ratios in the marketing of other substances; nevertheless, stable price increase is still highly recommended. Therefore, accompanying this policy should be more active measures for border control and for international cooperation to replace opium cultivation.

Note

1. Opium equivalent is the sum of heroin and morphine, which is equal to the amount of these substances multiplied by ten because ten grams of opium are required to produce one gram of heroin.

References

Annual opium poppy survey 2000. 2000. New York: Office for Drug Control and Crime Prevention, United Nations.

Annual report on the state of the drugs problem in the European Union. 2000. Brussels, Belgium: European Monitoring Center for Drugs and Drug Addiction.

Chearlo, Steffano. 1999. *Narcotics addiction in family relations.* Translated and compiled by Saeed Pirmoradi. Isfahan, Iran: Homan.

Community drug profile #1—Problem of drug use in Afghan communities: An initial assessment. 1999. Islamabad, Pakistan: Office for Drug Control and Crime Prevention, United Nations.

Community drug profile #2—Opium and other problem drug use in a group of Afghan refugee women. 1999. Islamabad, Pakistan: Office for Drug Control and Crime Prevention, United Nations.

Community drug profile #3—A comparative study of Afghan street heroin addicts in Peshawar and Quetta. 2000. Islamabad, Pakistan: Office for Drug Control and Crime Prevention, United Nations.

Dezhkam, Hossein. 2000. *Passage through the region 60° below zero.* Tehran, Iran: Porshokooh.

Doran-e Emrooz. 2001. *Etiad* (Addiction). 16 February.

Drug Control Headquarters (DCH). 1998. *Report of 1998.* Tehran: Drug Control Headquarters of Iran.

Drugs, money and laundering. 1998. Vienna: Office for Drug Control and Crime Prevention, United Nations.

Ghachagh-e Mavvad-e Makhader (Drug smuggling). 2000. *Bahar*, 19 July.

Global illicit drug trends 2000. 2000. New York: Office for Drug Control and Crime Prevention, United Nations.

Iran in the front line of drug battle: The national drug control report. 1999. Tehran: Islamic Republic of Iran.

Mahyar, Amir Houshang, and Mojtaba Jazayer. 1998. *Addiction, prevention and treatment*. Tehran, Iran: Ravan Pooya.

Masraf-e Mavvad-e Mokhader Dar Iran (Drug consumption in Iran). 2000. *Resalat*, 26 June.

Mavvad-e Mokhader (Drug). 2000. *Mosharekat*, 12 March.

Political declaration guiding principles of drug demand reduction and measures to enhance international cooperation to counter the world drug problem. 1999. Vienna: Office for Drug Control and Crime Prevention, United Nations.

Proceedings and papers of the seminar on issues relating to youth addiction. 1999. Tabriz, Iran: Office of the Governor of Tabriz.

Survey on drugs in Iran. 2000a. *Sobh Emrooz*, 23 February.

———. 2000b. *Sobh Emrooz*, 16 June.

State Welfare Organization of Islamic Republic of Iran. 1998. *Rehabilitation centers annual report*. Tehran: SWO of Iran.

———. 1999. *Rehabilitation centers annual report*. Tehran: SWO of Iran.

World drug report. 1997. United Nations, International Drug Control Programme, Oxford University Press.

The Price of Freedom:
Illegal Drug Markets and
Policies in Post-Soviet Russia

By LETIZIA PAOLI

ABSTRACT: In its difficult transition to democracy and a market economy, Russia has experienced a veritable boom of illegal markets, specifically the drug market. Drawing on the results of a study conducted on behalf of the United Nations, the first part of the article reconstructs the expansion of illegal drug consumption and trade in Russia since the collapse of the Soviet Union. It points, in particular, to the rapid diffusion of heroin, a substance that was virtually unknown in the former Soviet Union. The second part of the article reviews the measures taken by the Russian government to tackle illegal drug use and trafficking. It concludes that—as much as in the United States—the Russian drug policy is focused on supply reduction, whereas more funds and energies should be invested on the demand side for drug prevention, treatment, and harm reduction.

Letizia Paoli is a senior research fellow at the Department of Criminology of the Max Planck Institute for Foreign and International Criminal Law in Freiburg, Germany. She has published extensively on organized crime, drugs, and illegal markets. In the 1990s, she served as consultant to the Italian Ministries of the Interior and Justice, the UN Office for Drug Control and Crime Prevention, and the UN Crime and Justice Interregional Research Institute.

ONCE the core of the Soviet Empire, Russia has undergone a difficult transition to democracy and a market economy since 1991. Democratic political institutions were set up shortly after the collapse of the Soviet Union, but the full institutionalization of democracy is still hampered by weakness of the civil society and the limited autonomy of the media. The transition to a market economy has been even more difficult. In the 1990s, state enterprises were hastily privatized to former Soviet high-ranking officials' friends and cronies without previously setting up an institutional framework to ensure the proper functioning of the market. As a result, during the first ten years of the transition, a few robber barons rapidly accumulated enormous wealth, while Russia's GDP almost halved and the living conditions of the mainstream population worsened dramatically.

While the legal market economy has so far failed to fulfill its promises, the opening of borders and the liberalization of trade have triggered a veritable boom of illegal markets. In particular, since the collapse of the Soviet Union, a phenomenal expansion of illegal drug consumption and trade has taken place in Russia, as in most other countries of the former Warsaw Pact. Illegal psychoactive substances were used even prior to 1991, but during the Communist regime, both the number of consumers and the range of available substances were limited. Due to travel and trade restrictions, the former Soviet Union neither constituted a single drug market nor participated significantly in international narcotic exchanges as a consumer or supplier of illicit substances. However, this pattern of relative self-sufficiency drastically changed during the 1990s, as Russia rapidly became integrated in the international drug trade. Large quantities of illegal drugs today transit through the Russian territory to reach final consumers in Western and Eastern Europe. The growing domestic demand is also increasingly fed by more powerful and easier-to-use drugs imported from abroad. Besides expanding and tremendously diversifying its supply, the Russian drug market has, during the past ten years, become truly nationwide, and it now reaches even the remotest Siberian cities.

Since the fall of the Soviet Union, the Russian state authorities have responded in many ways to the expansion of illegal drug trade. Several program initiatives have been launched at both the domestic and international level; draconian sentencing provisions have been enacted to discourage drug dealing and trafficking. Despite these efforts, law enforcement agencies have been unable to prevent a near explosion in the scale of drug markets, while drug users and low-level dealers remain the primary target of their punitive action.

Several measures, among which is a new drug law, have also been passed to tackle the rapid increase of illegal drug use and abuse. Due to budget constraints, however, most of the demand-reduction initiatives foreseen by the new legislation have remained on paper, while most harm-reduction interventions are formally prohibited. As much as in the United States, the Russian drug policy is focused on supply reduction, whereas—according to many Russian and foreign observers—more funds and energies should be invested on the demand side for drug prevention, treatment, and harm reduction.

ILLEGAL DRUG USE AND TRADE IN THE TWILIGHT OF THE SOVIET REGIME

In some parts of Southern and Far Eastern Russia—and even more so, in the former Soviet Central Asian Republics—cannabis and poppies grow wild, and the use of these plants' derivatives has for centuries been ingrained in the local culture (Ministry of the Interior [MVD] 2000). In European Russia, where no such traditional consumption patterns are diffused, illegal drug use began to broaden in the late 1970s, most visibly among those nonconformist youth who were influenced by the U.S. hippie counterculture and who resorted to drugs to define their identity and to protest the constraints of the Soviet society. A second wave of expansion was registered in the late 1980s. Among the myriad of informal (*neformaly*) youth groups that developed "like mushrooms after the rain" in the wake of Gorbachev's *perestroika*, the regular or occasional use of illegal drugs became a frequent means of distinction (Pilkington 1994).

Only in the mid-1980s did the Soviet authorities begin to admit that their country—like the decadent capitalist societies—had a problem of drug abuse. According to a 1990 report of the Soviet MVD, the number of Soviet citizens "who had tried drugs or used them" totaled around 1.5 million (Lee 1992, 178). In ad hoc studies, academic scholars reached even higher estimates. In a school survey carried out in 1988-1989 among 5,801 secondary school students, 597 respondents, or 10.2 percent, admitted to taking illegal drugs. By extrapolation, the number of drug users among fourteen- to seventeen-year-old high school students was calculated at more than 1.5 million, and the total number of Soviet citizens who had taken drugs at least once in their lives was estimated at more than 15 million (Gabiani 1990). Whatever the true number of drug users in the Soviet Union, it is thus clear that the contemporary expansion of drug use has its roots in the Soviet era.

Up until the fall of the Soviet Union, in Russia as much as in the other Soviet republics, the largest part of the drug demand was supplied with locally produced substances. According to a second multiregional survey conducted by Anzor Gabiani in 1988-1989, among almost 3,000 regular and occasional drug users, the three most frequently used drugs nationwide were cannabis (whose derivatives, marijuana and hashish, were the first drugs of choice for 55 percent of the respondents), poppy straw, and opium (which were both selected by about 29 percent of the interviewees). Traditionally smoked, the latter two substances were usually processed by younger users into a strong solution of opioid alkaloids and then injected.

Chosen by 18 percent of the respondents, codeine, a synthetic opiate, was the fourth most popular drug (Gabiani 1990).

Due to the strict border control, imports represented a negligible share of the Soviet drug market, and even the domestic trade was rather limited because most people were not free to move. It is not by chance that the spread of the two drugs that are considered the most dangerous in the Western world (i.e., heroin and cocaine) was very low. Neither of them, in fact, was produced in the Soviet territory. As Rens Lee (1992) put it, up until the early 1990s, "the country [was] virtually self-sufficient in narcotics" (p. 184). This assessment is confirmed by the data gathered by the Drug Enforcement Division of the Soviet MVD: accordingly, 98 percent or more of the drugs consumed in the Soviet Union were of domestic origin (Lee 1992, 184).

"The Soviet narcotics market [was] highly imperfect by capitalist standards" (Lee 1992, 186). A developed drug distribution system hardly existed, and many users either produced or harvested their drugs themselves. Only a minority of consumers bought illicit psychoactive substances from a professional dealer (Gabiani 1990). Sophisticated production facilities for processing narcotics were relatively rare. Most manufactured drugs were home-made, usually prepared in the owner's own kitchen. Far from being managed by large-scale criminal organizations, most transfers and sales of drugs were carried out by individuals or small groups. It was predominantly a kind of "ants'

trafficking," which only rarely overcame the regional boundaries.

As no nationwide distribution system existed, drug consumption varied significantly by region and was largely dependent on the local availability of illegal psychoactive substances. People in the Northern European parts of the Soviet Union were far more likely to consume synthetic opiates and amphetamines than people in the Southern regions and the Far East, where plant-based substances were readily available (Gabiani 1990). Due to the bottlenecks in the Soviet drug distribution system, in some parts of the country, anesthetics with hallucinogen effects and toxic substances (such as glue, acetone, and gasoline) were also widely resorted to for lack of better alternatives (Paoli 2001b, 1-16).

THE DEMAND FOR
ILLEGAL DRUGS AFTER 1991

The disintegration of the Soviet Union and the difficult transition to democracy and a market economy have fostered the expansion of drug use and abuse in Russia since 1991. Even more than for their forerunners in the 1970s and 1980s, for contemporary Russian urban youth, illegal drugs have become a means to demonstrate their assimilation to Western lifestyles and to display their newly obtained freedom of action.

Drug use also reflects the lack of orientation suffered by many Russian teenagers and young adults. In a society that has abandoned its old value system and has not yet established a new one, young people recognize neither their parents nor their teachers as role models. They tend to consider older people's values, lifestyles, and experiences meaningless and without any practical significance. As Igor Ilynsky (1995), the rector of the Institute of Youth Studies in Moscow, stated, the Russian society is not merely experiencing the usual "generation conflict," entailing different opinions on dress, hairstyle, music, dance, and behavior. "Russian society is actually facing . . . a *break in generations* reflecting a rupture of continuity, a rupture in historical development, a transition of society to a principally different economic, social and political system" (p. 106). In such a phase of rupture, drugs have become an accessible means to express youth opposition to older generations' models and one's willingness to go one's own way, radically departing from standard life paths.

For a small but rapidly growing minority of Russian youth, moreover, drugs increasingly represent what Robert Merton (1949) called the "retreatist adaptation": that is, the rejection of the dominant cultural goals and institutional means. Unable to reach the glamorous aims of a society for which wealth is becoming the primary and exclusive measure of people's value, young Russians increasingly resort to illegal drugs to escape their harsh living conditions, to forget their broken dreams, and to cope with unemployment and marginalization.

The Russian MVD estimates that 2.5 to 3 million people in the Russian Federation regularly or occasionally use illegal drugs, which represents 2.1 percent of the total population (United Nations Office for Drug Control and Crime Prevention [UNODCCP] 2001). In absolute values, this figure is not staggering. In 1999 in the United States, for comparison, 14.8 million Americans (5.4 percent of the population) reported using an illicit drug at least once during the thirty days prior to the interview (Substance Abuse and Mental Health Services Administration 2000). What makes Russia's case so astounding is the sudden growth in drug use and, above all, drug abuse. The abrupt expansion of these phenomena is clearly shown in the data regarding drug users who were registered for the first time in state drug treatment centers. In 1991, 3.9 cases per 100,000 inhabitants were recorded yearly. In the following years, there has been a veritable escalation, and in 1999, there were 42 cases per 100,000 inhabitants. The Ministry of Health estimates that the number of drug users for the first time entering treatment would have reached the rate of 48.5 per 100,000 people by the end of the year 2000 (UNODCCP 2001, 8).

Though cannabis remains the most frequently used illegal drug in Russia as in most other countries, heroin consumption has rapidly increased. The latter substance started to be available in Moscow and other Russian cities in the mid-1990s and rapidly became a substitute for the less powerful homemade opiates that were previously injected by Russian users. Today, heroin attracts not only intravenous drug addicts, but also teenagers from all social backgrounds who initially smoke it, although many of them end up injecting it. Six percent of fifteen- to sixteen-year-old high school students interviewed in Moscow in 1999 admitted to having used heroin at least once in their lives. In none of the twenty-one other countries involved in the European Project of School Research in Alcohol and Drug Use survey did the lifetime prevalence rate exceed 2 percent (Vishinsky 1999).

While heroin became widespread in Russia only in the late 1990s, the high prevalence of heroin use among Russian high school students points to a larger trend: the spread of injecting drug use among teenagers and young adults. In Western Europe, injecting drug use is commonly widespread among low-class marginalized young and, increasingly, not so young people. In Russia, on the other hand, a straightforward association as such cannot be made; rather drug use, including intravenous drug use, seems to involve youth from all social classes and ethnic groups (Paoli 2001b, 17-20; Gilinsky, Kostjukovsky, and Rusakova 2000, 15).

In the late 1990s, injecting use of heroin and other drugs was shown to be an alarming means of spreading HIV and AIDS. The World Health Organization (Wines 1999) recently reported "an explosive increase in HIV infections" in Russia. In 2000, 46,438 cases of HIV infections were identified. This is almost twice the total of 29,000 infections recorded in the country between 1987 and 1999. However, even this massive rise understates the real growth of the epidemic. By Russian estimates, the national registration system captures just a fraction of the infections. According to conservative forecasts, more than 1 million people could be infected with HIV by the end of 2001 (UNODCCP 2001, 9, 18).

THE RISE OF A NATIONWIDE MARKET FOR ILLEGAL DRUGS

The Russian drug market tremendously expanded its turnover in the 1900s, as seizure data (though indirectly) prove. During the last decade of the twentieth century, in fact, the amount of illicit drugs confiscated by the Russian MVD grew 3.5 times, from 16,260 kilograms in 1990 to 59,343 kilograms in 1999. Even more spectacular has been the rise of heroin seizures: this substance was largely unknown until 1992, when only 5 grams were intercepted in all of Russia. Since then, heroin seizures have increased continuously, reaching 984 kilograms in 2000 (UNODCCP 2001).

The expansion of the Russian illegal drug market has affected not only its turnover but also its geographic extent. Most illicit drugs are currently available in virtually all Russian regions, and supplying oneself with various kinds of illicit drugs has become easier in all Russian cities. In St. Petersburg (Russia's second largest city), according to a young consumer, "you have the impression that you can buy drugs everywhere" (Gilinsky, Kostjukovsky, and Rusakova 2000, 21). The growing drug availability involves not only the metropolises but also the middle and smaller centers, where the changes may possibly have been even more spectacular (see, e.g., Markoryan 2000). To get their high or forget their sorrows, drug users all over Russia are no longer obliged to rely on toxic substances, homemade products, or derivatives of locally grown plants. If they can afford it, users can easily purchase the same illicit psychoactive drugs that can be found in any Western European or North American city, imported from countries as far away as Colombia, Afghanistan, and Holland. Although cannabis has retained its predominance, there also has been a shift from plant extracts and homemade solutions to ready-to-use preparations.

Heroin is imported—via the former Soviet Central Asian Republics—from Afghanistan, the source of two-thirds to three-quarters of the global supply of illicit opiates in recent years. Former Soviet communication routes are increasingly exploited, not only to satisfy the growing domestic demand, but also to smuggle heroin into Europe. Following the loosening of border controls and the liberalization of trade, other illegal drugs, such as cocaine and ecstasy, have also become available in Russia. The former is imported either directly from Latin America or, more frequently, from Western European countries; the latter is predominantly smuggled from Holland (Paoli 2001b, 74-90). Whereas ecstasy is becoming popular among young people of all social strata, cocaine is still consumed—due to its prohibitive prices—only by a tiny minority of "new Russians," the sole ones who can afford it (Paoli 2001b, 60-63).

THE "INVISIBLE HAND" OF THE MARKET

The growth of Russian drug consumption and trade in the 1990s entailed the emergence of a nationwide drug distribution system, delivering illicit drugs from producers to consumers thanks to the mediation of full-time or part-time traffickers and dealers. The latter roles did not exist in Russia prior to the early 1990s, comparable to the situation in Western Europe and the United States up until the mid-1970s. It was not until the drug supply diversified and Russia entered into international drug trade that the drug distributor, as a professional role, emerged to link producers to consumers and to regularly supply large urban centers with a variety of illegal drugs from distant regions.

In official reports, Russian law enforcement authorities present a very "organized" picture of the drug trade. In its latest report on drug and organized crime, for example, the MVD (2000) categorically stated that "drug crime is always organized" (p. 5). The idea that drug trafficking is dominated by large, structured criminal groups finds, however, scarce support even in law enforcement statistical data. It is enough to say that the crimes committed by "organized crime groups" represent less than 1 percent of the total drug offences reported in Russia during the 1990s and in 1999 accounted for only 4.1 percent of drug trafficking cases (Paoli 2001b, 91-93).

No proof of large-scale trafficking organizations emerges from the fifty-two drug-related criminal proceedings that were analyzed by the author together with the Research Institute of the Prosecutor General's Office (Paoli 2001a). Although the defendants frequently received draconian sentences because they were suspected of belonging to an organized group, the existence of such groups remained largely unproved. In the Russian jurisprudence, in fact, a drug transaction between the buyer and the seller or even the common purchase of illegal drugs by two users are considered sufficient to apply the organized crime group aggravating circumstances. And this assumption holds even when the other components of the group remain unknown: in thirty-six of the analyzed cases, there was only one defendant. Likewise, although aggravating circumstances due to the extremely large scale of the confiscated drugs were often applied, in most cases, the amounts were minimal, at least according to Western standards. Defendants were sentenced to more than five years of imprisonment, for buying and partially selling drug amounts ranging from 3.3 milliliters of *vint*,[1] 0.15 and 0.17 grams of opium, and 0.091 and 0.0058 grams of heroin.

The relatively "disorganized" (Reuter 1983) nature of drug trafficking and distribution in Russia is further shown by the fieldwork conducted in nine Russian cities (including Moscow, St. Petersburg, Nizhniy Novgorod, Krasnoyarsk, and Vladivostok) on behalf of the UNODCCP (Paoli 2001b). The UN-sponsored project could indeed prove that a multilevel drug distribution system had developed in all of these cities, which led to users'

increasingly buying drugs from dealers instead of cultivating or harvesting them themselves. The consumers' demands, however, seem to be neither satisfied nor promoted by the large, hierarchically organized firms that monopolize local markets.

The phenomenal growth of drug use can thus be attributed to the invisible hand of the market: the local drug markets of Russian cities are today largely supplied by a myriad of drug dealers who tend to operate alone or in small groups and often consume illegal drugs themselves. In many cases, the dealers do not possess previous criminal expertise and deal with illegal drugs simply to earn a living or to supplement the meager income they obtain from licit activities. As a Moscow police officer put it,

There are no Colombian drug cartels here. There are instead many small groups that are made of people belonging to the same nationality or ethnic group. There is not one single river, but many streams that flow independently on one another. (Paoli 2001b, 102)

Although the members of some ethnic communities (above all, Roma, Tajik, Afghani, and Azeri) may be overproportionally represented in the drug distribution system of many Russian cities, illegal drugs are also produced and sold by many people belonging to the mainstream Russian population who cannot be precisely classified. As Ludmila Markoryan (2000) from Balakovo (a Southern Russian city close to the border with Kazakhstan) pointed out,

It is not easy to refer the drug dealers of our city to specific social groups. Dealer might be a housewife, a jobless person, or a businessman. The age range of middle and high-ranking drug dealers also varies tremendously: there are young people as well as retirees.

COUNTERNARCOTIC OPERATIONS: RHETORIC AND PRACTICES

In its philosophy and goals, the drug policy of the Russian Federation presents a strong continuity with that pursued by the former Soviet Union: not only do they aim at a drug-free world but they regard repression and coercion as legitimate means to curb both the consumption and the traffic of illegal drugs. What has changed during the past ten years is the amount of human and material resources that are invested in the fight against illegal drugs. Previously ranked as a secondary task, since 1991, counternarcotic operations have become one of the most important and prestigious activities for all Russian law enforcement agencies. These have frequently exploited the fight against drug abuse and trade to justify their existence as well as their growing funding needs, and ever since the early 1990s, reforms were passed to adjust to the new tasks. In 1991, the Drug Control Department was set up within the MVD, and in less than a decade, its staff more than tripled, exceeding five thousand units. In the following years, similar entities were set up within other law enforcement agencies: in the State Customs Committee, the Federal Security Service (the former KGB), and the Federal Border Guards (MVD 1999, 28-30).

As the cooperation among these bodies has not always been smooth and effective, in May 1998, the Interagency Drug Control Center was established, which is composed of officials of the above-mentioned bodies and is attached to the MVD. According to several interviewees, however, even the work of the Interagency Drug Control Center is hampered by persisting rivalries among the various law enforcement agencies and among departments of the MVD itself (Paoli 2001b, 128-34).

Since the fall of the Soviet Union, considerable efforts were made to intensify Russia's cooperation with international organizations and foreign countries on drug control matters. Besides working more closely with the UNODCCP, in May 1999, the Russian Federation became a member of the Council of Europe Co-operation Group to Combat Drug Abuse and the Illicit Trafficking in Drugs (the so-called Pompidou Group). Bilateral and multilateral cooperation has also increased rapidly since the early 1990s. As of November 1999, more than eighty intergovernmental and interagency agreements with fifty-seven states had been concluded, which fully or partially deal with drug control cooperation. Working contracts were also established with a number of countries with which bilateral agreements had not been concluded (MVD 2000, 39-43).

On the basis of the above agreements, since the early 1990s, Russian law enforcement agencies carried out numerous counternarcotic operations together with their counterparts in foreign countries. In the late

1990s, the former were involved in about 150 international drug-controlled deliveries (MVD 2000, 39-43). In particular, to hamper the heroin trade, since 1993, the Russian Federal Border Guards have been patrolling the border between Afghanistan and Tajikistan, seizing more than three thousand kilograms of heroin in 2000 (UNODCCP 2001, 17). Aside from Tajikistan, however, mistrust and suspicion often pollute joint operations with the law enforcement agencies of former Soviet republics. Almost ironically, according to Russian and foreign police officers alike, the counternarcotic cooperation seems to be the smoothest with the Western countries, which were Russia's main enemy up to a decade ago (Paoli 2001b, 132-34).

Reflecting the larger resources invested in counternarcotics operations, both the number of seizures and the amounts of confiscated drugs increased tremendously during the 1990s. Even the number of reported drug offences grew spectacularly from 16,255 in 1990 to 216,364 in 1999. By analyzing the latter statistical data, however, it becomes clear that—despite official rhetoric—drug users are the main target of state counternarcotic efforts. On average, in fact, between 1990 and 1999, more than 77 percent of all registered drug offences involved the mere possession of very small drug quantities without the purpose of sale (Paoli 2001b, 134-39).

As a matter of fact, according to the 1996 Russian Criminal Code, the possession of narcotics "not on a large scale" is considered a mere adminis-

trative infraction and not a criminal offence (Ciklauri-Lammich 2001). Only if drug users are caught with large-scale amounts of drugs are they prosecuted, pursuant to article 228, paragraph 1, for the "acquisition and keeping without the purpose of sale of narcotic drugs," which is punishable with imprisonment up to three years. The amounts set by the Standing Committee on Narcotic Drug Control of the Russian Ministry of Health to establish the meaning of "large scale" are, however, so low that most consumers, even if they are found with minimal quantities of drugs, exceed them. According to the table published by the Standing Committee in December 1998, in fact, "not large scale" amounts are considered to be the following:

- hashish: up to 0.1 gram
- dried marijuana: up to 0.1 gram
- not dried marijuana: up to 0.5 gram
- opium: up to 0.1 gram
- morphine: up to 0.1 gram. (Standing Committee on Narcotic Drug Control 1999)

To avoid the explicit decriminalization of the acquisition and possession of even very small amounts, the commission set no figure for heavy drugs and specifically for heroin. In agreement with the Supreme Court and the prosecutor's office, the Russian MVD subsequently issued a recommendation in which it stated that a criminal case can be opened only if a "portion" of illegal drugs capable of producing psychoactive effects on its user was seized (Paoli 2001b, 124). The notion of portion is, however, very conservatively interpreted, and a few milligrams of heroin are usually enough to open a penal proceeding for the acquisition and possession of drugs on a large scale. In the Russian jurisprudence, in fact, more than 0.005 grams of heroin and more than 0.0001 grams of LSD are usually considered large amounts (Gilinsky, Kostjukovsky, and Rusakova 2000, 32). Indeed, as the above-mentioned analysis of drug-related crime proceedings demonstrates, even the prosecution of more serious offences overwhelmingly targets drug users. It is thus fair to conclude that most of the persons who are arrested and prosecuted yearly in Russia for drug offences are not dealers but users.

The only way to avoid falling into the law enforcement net is to bribe police officers: this is—according to many drug users, dealers, and even police officers themselves—by no means an infrequent practice. Throughout Russia, in fact, many patrol officers accept—and frequently even extort—bribes from drug users and dealers to supplement their meager wages (a Russian police officer earns less than 100 dollars a month) or to cope with the sometimes lengthy wage arrears (Paoli 2001b, 64-67). As a drug user–dealer in St. Petersburg maintained,

If I have to describe all the occasions I gave money to the police, it is going to become a lengthy volume. If I am arrested when I have money or drugs, I always pay. If I have no money, I call my girlfriend or some other friend by mobile phone to come and help me. (Gilinsky, Kostjukovsky, and Rusakova 2000, 31-32)

THE NEGLECT OF DEMAND AND HARM-REDUCTION STRATEGIES

The development of treatment and rehabilitation institutions constitutes one of the main priorities set by the Federal Law on Narcotic Drugs and Psychotropic Substances, which was approved on 10 December 1997. According to its article 54, in fact, "the state guarantees help to drug addicts, including examination, consulting, diagnostics, treatment, and social-medical rehabilitation." Most of these services are supposed to be freely and exclusively provided by public hospitals and day care centers because the new legislation explicitly sets a state monopoly on treatment (article 55).

The state drug treatment centers, however, do not have the financial, material, and human resources to fulfill the tasks that are assigned them by the law. Due to budget constraints, a specific bill concerning the "social and medical help for drug addicts," which was to complete the federal drug law, has never been issued. As a result, even in public health institutions, most drug users have to pay for services that should have been obtained gratis. Moreover, for fear of being reported to the police, many users do not willingly turn to state drug treatment centers for help—with the paradoxical consequence that these often operate below their restricted capacities.

The shortcomings of state drug treatment centers are only partially offset by the private ones. These formally operate *contra legem* but are present in virtually all Russian cities, and in some contexts they even advertise in newspapers (Paoli

2001b, 139-41). Private centers are, above all, popular because they offer the guarantee of anonymous treatment. They represent, however, a viable alternative only for those users coming from rich families who can afford to pay up to U.S.$200 a day.

The new drug law also sets a state monopoly on drug prevention activities—but only a handful of the eighty-nine subjects of the Russian Federation have so far found the money to carry out large-scale drug prevention and information campaigns. As in the case of treatment, the formal prohibition is often disregarded, and some of the gaps left by federal and state bodies are filled by Russian and foreign nongovernmental organizations. In several areas, these have launched harm-reduction projects to inform users about the risks associated with drug use and teach them risk-reduction techniques. Thanks to the financial support of George Soros's Open Society Institute and the training and technical assistance of Médecins sans Frontières, for example, peer-driven intervention and needle exchange programs were started in the late 1990s in more than twenty Russian cities. Though these programs have the approval of the local city and regional administrations, many of their coordinators report interference by the police and resent working on the fringe of legality (Sergeyev et al. 1999; Burrows et al. 2000).

As harm-reduction measures are one of the few effective means to reduce the spread of HIV, many Russian and foreign, public and private drug-treatment providers call for their intensification and full legalization (Paoli 2001b, 141). These observers also insist that demand and harm-reduction strategies should be granted at least the same relevance and financial, human, and material resources as are invested in repression activities. At least in the short term, however, there seems to be no reason to expect a radical shift in the Russian drug policy, as both the general public and the law enforcement agencies (including the powerful MVD) support a tough and uncompromising stance vis-à-vis both drug dealers and users. Only the coming explosion of HIV infections may perhaps legitimize harm-reduction measures and trigger a paradigm change—as happened under analogous circumstances in several Western European countries in the late 1980s and early 1990s.

No matter what the drug policy emphasis will be, there is no doubt that Russia will have to learn to cope with extensive illegal drug consumption and trade in the near future. As in Central and Eastern Europe, the post-Soviet transition to democracy and a market economy have given the Russian people an unprecedented degree of freedom—including that of buying illegal drugs as long as they can afford to. The excepted high profits from the illegal drug trade and the dire living conditions of most Russians ensure that the domestic demand for illegal drugs will go on being met—and, to some extent, even fostered by importers and distributors. Finally, due to its geographical position, Russia will certainly go on being crossed by heroin cargos on their way to the rich consumer markets in Western Europe, at least as long as Afghanistan remains one of the largest world opium and heroin producers. Even though many Russian citizens are shocked to realize it, the recent expansion of the illegal drug market constitutes a reliable—though worrying—indicator of the long way they have gone since 1991.

Note

1. Vint is a methamphetamine solution that can be produced domestically by the users themselves and that was very popular in Russia in the late 1980s and early 1990s.

References

Burrows, D., F. Trautmann, M. Bijl, and Y. Sarankov. 2000. Training in the Russian Federation on rapid assessment and response to HIV/AIDS among injecting drug users. *Journal of Drug Issues* (fall): 811-41.

Ciklauri-Lammich, E. 2001. Das russische Betäubungsmittelrecht unter besonderer Berücksichtigung der strafrechtlichen Regelung. *Jahrbuch für Ostrecht* 42:12-29.

Gabiani, A. A. 1990. Narkotism v zerkalye sotsiologii (Narcotism in the mirror of sociology). Unpublished manuscript.

Gilinsky, Y., Y. Kostjukovsky, and M. Rusakova. 2000. Site report on drug markets, drug trafficking, and organized crime in St. Petersburg. Unpublished manuscript.

Ilynsky, I. 1995. The spiritual and cultural values of young people on a post-totalitarian state. In *Young people in post-Communist Russia and Eastern Europe*, edited by J. Riordan, C. Williams, and I. Ilynsky, 97-115. Aldershot, UK: Dartmouth.

Lee, R. 1992. Dynamics of the Soviet illicit drug market. *Crime, Law and Social Change* 17:177-233.

Markoryan, L. 2000. Potreblenije i torgovla narkotikami v Balakovo (Drug use and drug trafficking in Balakovo). Unpublished manuscript.

Merton, R. 1949. *Social theory and social structure*. New York: Free Press.

Ministry of the Interior (MVD). 1999. *Drug situation in Russian Federation*. Moscow: Ministry of the Interior.

———. 2000. *Kontrol sa narkotikami i predypresdenie prestypnosti v Rossijskoj Federazii: Organisovannaja prestypnost i nesakonnij oborot narkotikov v Rossijskoj Federazii* (Drug control and crime prevention in the Russian Federation: Organized crime and illicit drug trafficking in the Russian Federation). Moscow: Ministry of the Interior.

Paoli, L. 2001a. Drug trafficking in Russia: A form of organized crime? *Journal of Drug Issues* 31 (4): 1005-34.

———. 2001b. *Illegal drug trade in Russia: A research project commissioned by the United Nations Office for Drug Control and Crime Prevention*. Freiburg, Germany: Edition Iuscrim.

Pilkington, H. 1994. *Russia's youth and its culture. A nation's constructors and constructed*. London: Routledge.

Reuter, P. 1983. *Disorganized crime: The economics of the visible hand*. Cambridge, MA: MIT Press.

Sergeyev, B., T. Oparina, T. P. Rumyantseva, V. L. Volkanevskii, R. S. Broadhead, D. D. Heckathorn, and H. Madray. 1999. HIV-prevention in Yaroslavl, Russia: A peer-driven intervention and needle exchange. *Journal of Drug Issues* 29 (3): 777-804.

Standing Committee on Narcotic Drug Control. 1999. Svodnaja Tablica zaklucenij postojannego komiteta po kontroliu narkotikov ob otnnesenii k nebolsim, krupnym i osobo krupnym razmieram kolicestv narkoticeskich sredstv, psychotropnych i silnodiejstvujuscich vescestv, obnaruzennych v nezakonnom chranieni ili oborotie (Note to the table summarizing the decisions of the Standing Committee for Drug Control concerning small, large, and especially large amounts of narcotic drugs, psychotropic substances, and other psychoactive substances, which were detected in cases of illegal possession and sale). *Bjuletin Verchovnego Suda Rossiskoj Federacji* 4:15-19.

Substance Abuse and Mental Health Services Administration, U.S. Department of Health and Human Services. 2000. *1999 National Household Survey on Drug Abuse.* Retrieved from http://www.SAMHSA.gov/household99.htm.

United Nations Office for Drug Control and Crime Prevention (UNODCCP), Regional Office for Russia and Belarus. 2001. *Annual field report 2000 Russia.* Retrieved from http://www.undcp.org/russia/report_2000-12-31_1.html

Vishinsky, K. 1999. *Isytshenije rasprostranennosti ypotreblenija psixoaktivnix veshestv na primere goroda Moskvi* (Analysis of the spread of psychotropic substances in Russia and specifically in Moscow). Moscow: Scientific Research Institute of Narcology, Ministry of Health.

Wines, M. 1999. Needle use sets off HIV explosion in Russia. *New York Times,* 24 November.

ANNALS, *AAPSS*, **582**, July 2002

Money Laundering
and Its Regulation

By MICHAEL LEVI

ABSTRACT: This article examines definitions of "money laundering" and the conceptual and actual role its regulation plays in dealing with drug markets. If laundering is prevented, incentives to become major criminals are diminished. It identifies and critiques three aspects of harm arising from laundering: facilitating crime groups' expansion, corroding financial institutions, and extent. After a discussion of laundering techniques used with drug money, including the symbiotic relationship with some otherwise legitimate ordinary businesses, the article examines the history of public- and private-sector antilaundering policies and their implementation in the United States and globally. It concludes that much detected laundering involves the same out-of-place judgments the police use, but though the proportion of routine and suspicious activity reports that yield arrests may be low, they do generate some important enforcement actions. Nevertheless, the impact of antilaundering efforts on enforcement resources, organized crime markets, or drug consumption levels remains modestly understood at present.

Dr. Michael Levi is a professor of criminology at Cardiff University, Wales. His major research contributions have been in the fields of white-collar crime and corruption, organized crime, money laundering, and violent crime, and he is a scientific expert on organized crime to the Council of Europe and the European Union. His book Victims of White-Collar Crime *will be published by Clarendon Press in 2002. He is currently completing a study of policy development and transfer in the area of money laundering, corruption, and asset forfeiture funded by the U.K. Economic and Social Research Council's Future Governance Research Initiative.*

"**M**ONEY laundering," like "organized crime," is one of those terms of both criminological and popular discourse that evokes images of sophisticated multinational financial operations that transform proceeds of drug trafficking into clean money. National legislation in many parts of the world (as well as international instruments) typically began by criminalizing the laundering of the proceeds of drug trafficking before, perhaps some years later, broadening the scope to include all or most serious crimes (tax evasion being the key area of dispute).[1] This reflects the evolution of thinking about the logic of antilaundering policies (discussed later) as well as the pragmatic politics of legislating what the political market will bear: getting international consensus is easier for dealing with drug trafficking than with corruption, environmental crime, tax evasion or—at least prior to the carnage of 11 September 2001—terrorism. It is now only on tax cooperation issues that a significant constituency of bankers or politicians is prepared nowadays to assert publicly that preserving financial privacy is much more important than fighting the menace of serious crimes such as drug and human trafficking. What was formerly a genteel sovereign right of any nation to ensure "customer confidentiality" has become redefined pejoratively as unacceptable "bank secrecy" that facilitates the drug trade (Levi 1991). In this global risk management process, modern areas of law enforcement have sought to free themselves from the constraints of due process and similar old-fashioned ideas of protection against overzealous state intrusions by focusing on disruption and on situational strategic laundering prevention.

The United States is atypical in its early imposition of tough measures against organized crime generally, for example, the Racketeer Influenced and Corrupt Organizations (RICO) Act of 1970. The range of its application soon broadened, as is illustrated by the use of RICO against targets as varied as corrupt labor unions, Italian American syndicate stock manipulation, and alleged oil sanctions busting by Marc Rich and associates. To this was added, from 1986, legislation against money laundering.[2]

What is money laundering and why is it important? In essence, it encompasses any concealing of the proceeds of drug trafficking (or other serious crimes) beyond putting the loot visibly on the bed or in one's domestic safe. If the opportunity to pretend that one's wealth is legitimate—if and when challenged—can be effectively denied, then the motivation for continued crime and the political/social threat from rich criminals is considerably reduced. The logic of controlling the drug money trail is that profit motivates drug sales, and because most sales—certainly at street level—are (or are believed to be) in cash, the recipient of cash has to find some way of converting these funds into utilizable financial resources that appear to have legitimate origins. If they are prevented from doing so, their incentives to become major criminals are diminished, so there is both a general and a specific threshold preventative effect from antilaundering efforts. These preventative effects can be reinforced by (1) requirements on financial and other risk-prone institutions to report large cash and/or suspicious transactions to specialized police or administrative intelligence units and (2) proceeds of crime confiscation or forfeiture laws that are intended to incapacitate both individuals and criminal organizations from accumulating substantial criminal capital and the socioeconomic power that accrues from this.

The Financial Action Task Force (FATF) was created by G-7 in 1989 as a temporary working group to develop measures to implement antilaundering policies. It has a small secretariat (colocated with the Organization for Economic Cooperation and Development) and twenty-nine governmental members (plus the European Commission and the Gulf Co-operation Council). The FATF has described laundering as a three-stage process: the placement of funds into the financial system; the layering of funds to disguise their origin, perhaps by passing through several offshore and/or onshore jurisdictions; and the integration of the funds into the legitimate economy. Cash is less often used for placement in fraud and grand corruption (i.e., high-level public officials) cases and in sophisticated forms of extortion in which inflated prices are paid for services than it is used for drugs, which have a more elaborate sales distribution network. In the case of terrorism, most living expenses and purchases can be paid for in cash, which leaves little paper trail.

The need to prove a specific predicate offence before convicting for laundering varies between countries. Many common law jurisdictions and an increasing number of civil law ones have criminalized "own funds laundering," so that if a local drug dealer walks into his or her local bank with a modest $100 in bills and deposits the cash in his or her bank account in his or her own name, he or she commits the offense of money laundering (if it can be proven that these are proceeds of a crime). This—most common in the United States and Belgium—is regarded by some European scholars as a legal abomination since it can lead to two charges for the same act (Stessens 2000); it also leads to the same legal category's being used for these simple acts and for global financial chicanery using offshore havens, making comparative analysis difficult.[3]

Laundering can be considered important for three reasons:

1.   It facilitates crime by capacitating crime groups and networks to self-finance, diversify, and grow.

2.   It can have a corrosive impact on financial institutions and other parties. However, there is an element of paradox here. For centuries, onshore and offshore bankers have been tolerantly laundering proceeds of many crimes and from many countries without obvious harm to them or to their economies. Criminal (as opposed to moral) corruption of bankers and trust/company formation agents in some jurisdictions has been made necessary as a consequence of the criminalization of laundering and of regulations intended to stop

willful blindness. Given those regulations, laundering can be harmful to the financial system of laundering countries and creates serious reputational risk irrespective of the impacts on domestic crime there. In the Third World (including the former Soviet Union), the issues are more complex. Their economies vitally need investment capital, and if launderers provided venture capital without eliminating indigenous people from this function (economically and/or physically), then this might not be harmful. However, in practice, criminal funds can be used to create a license to operate piratically in a hollow state rather than for productive purposes, and criminally owned banks created to launder funds can also be used to defraud the public (though to do so will terminate their usefulness as laundering vehicles since normally they will close down as a result).

3. A third measure of harm is the extent of laundering, though this depends on which crimes are included and on harm to legitimate capital; unfortunately, there is no consensus on what this is. Figures of $300 billion to $500 billion for international flows are banded around and become "facts by repetition," but there is very little evidence to justify them (van Duyne 1998; van Duyne and de Miranda 1999). For an FATF exercise that ended in fundamental disagreement, Walker (1999) heroically attempted to construct money flows into all-crime and drug laundering guesstimation exercises, while Reuter (2000) made a sophisticated attempt to construct global expenditure on drugs as the sum of national estimates; outside the United States, national expenditure data are deeply unreliable, and even in the United States, the range is a broad $40 billion to $100 billion. Moreover, money laundered in year 1 may have to be relaundered in year 2, when it may have to be invested. Finally, criminal business costs (including protection and salaries to terrorist or crime gang members) and lifestyle expenditures—both high in multilayered drug business—have to be subtracted from the crime proceeds data before we reach the laundering figures, which are anyway dependent on the savings ratios of offenders. (Part of the business costs take the form of income for others and flow directly into the GNP.)

If drug dealers retain property of value, whether or not traceable directly to crime, they may need to launder to enable them to account for possessions they cannot justify by officially earned income and wealth if they live in places that have civil forfeiture regimes (in the United States and Ireland, and shortly in the UK, for example) or—if they can be convicted—the many criminal confiscation/forfeiture laws that reverse the onus of proof postconviction.

How is money laundered? Laundering needs to be only good enough to defeat the changing capacity of financial investigation skills and burden of proof in any of the jurisdictions along its economic path. Devices such as "walking trust accounts"—which move automatically to another jurisdiction when inquiries or mutual assistance requests are made in one jurisdiction—clearly act as facilitators of crime and inhibitors of responses by making it very much more expensive, if indeed possible at all, to pursue the defendants either for evidence or for recompense. But only the most sophisticated end of the laundering trade uses these. The *World Drug Report* (United Nations International Drug Control Programme 1997, 138 *et seq.*) sets out some techniques:

1. "Smurfing" is a process whereby "the cash is exchanged for bearer cheques or international money orders, which are then deposited into the trafficker's account by an intermediary of the same organization. . . . In most cases [smurfs] need know nothing beyond the amount of cash they are required to convert and their fee."[4]

2. "The use of cash-intensive businesses in money-laundering is extremely prevalent."

3. There are accounting techniques under which the difference between the artificially high invoice price and the real price of the goods and services is deposited offshore. These are used also by those who wish to avoid taxes and duties.

4. There are private investment techniques, including "loan backs," where the launderer makes an investment with a loan secured on his offshore funds, which is then repaid.

5. There is the use of nonbank financial institutions, such as cashing in large single premium payments, getting a refund on part-used plane tickets, and cashing in casino chips.

6. There is investment in government bonds as bearer instruments, presumably for cash.

7. There is the opportunistic lending/acquisition of companies on the verge of bankruptcy.

8. There is the exploitation of underground banking systems.

However, the extent to which these are used for drug money, and by traffickers at what levels, is not mapped out with any clarity. More helpful is the analysis found in a review of money laundering and its control conducted for the United Nations the following year (Blum et al. 1998), which illustrates the use of trusts, international business corporations, and free trade zones for laundering schemes, indicating also that proceeds of drug sales in the United States and elsewhere can be used by Third World businesspeople to avoid exchange control restrictions in their home countries (in what is known as the "black peso market"). A sanitized version of money-laundering typologies is available from the FATF periodically. (For some interesting data and general reflections on black markets and "extralegality" in the Third World, see de Soto 2000.)

MONEY-LAUNDERING AND
ANTICRIME STRATEGIES

Proactive anti-drug-trafficking methods cannot plausibly prevent all smuggling. Therefore, the attempt to monitor financial transactions and confiscate crime proceeds is the obvious next key strategy in the organized crime containment program (see, e.g., Office of National Drug Control Strategy 2001). This requires a major global infrastructure of compatible legislation and mutual legal assistance both for financial investigation and for proceeds of crime restraint and confiscation. The United States, supported from the start by Australia, France, and the United Kingdom, was the principal enthusiast for antilaundering measures to attack kingpins of the drug trade but, as Gilmore (1999) has observed, the rapidity (less than two years) with which the 1988 UN Vienna Convention came into force is testimony to the power of drug issues in the political culture of nations around the world. What effects it has had on the availability, production, and distribution of illegal drugs remains doubtful. Nevertheless, there has been continued reform of antilaundering and crime proceeds legislation around the world (Gilmore 1999; Levi 1997, 2001; Stessens 2000) and greater policing (including customs and excise) involvement in financial investigation, still mainly in the drug field but increasingly in excise tax fraud and, post-2001, terrorism. The Egmont Group of Financial Investigation Units that ensures some cross-national cooperation has developed substantially since the mid-1990s, though its practical effects have not been evaluated properly. With the targeting of persons rather than simply activities in offender risk management strategies (Maguire 2000), the precise context in which prosecutions and asset confiscation occur has become flexible.

Particularly since 1996, FATF and its regional associates in different parts of the world (starting with the Caribbean and expanding to include Asia Pacific and Latin America, with Africa developing a regional body), alongside the Council of Europe, the European Union, and the United Nations, have moved away from the initial exclusive drug focus in antilaundering policy toward an all-crime and transnational organized crime focus, though the effects of this are not obvious since, as Levi (1991) and Gold and Levi (1994) observed in their studies of how suspicious financial transaction reports come to be constructed and followed through, few bankers know in what types of crime—if any—their customers may be engaged. As I write in mid-2001, FATF member states are far from agreement over whether countries should be compelled to include tax offenses as a predicate for money laundering.

The slow adoption of FATF standards in some territories—many of whom are not members of key bodies and have not been evaluated by peers—precipitated the Non Cooperating Countries and Territories initiative commenced in 2000. This economically blacklists the (fifteen in the first tranche, with some changes in the second) countries "named and shamed." This blacklisting is accompanied by treasury advisories to all regulated banks telling them that they should exercise special care in dealing with transactions from the named jurisdictions, with more severe sanctions in prospect for persistent noncompliance. Conformity to these directives also becomes part of the banks' compliance audit. There is no provision to appeal against blacklisting, which has been criticized for picking on non–member states while tolerating some similar malpractices among member states.

APPROACHES TO MONEY-LAUNDERING REGULATION

At the level of the nation-state, there are essentially two sorts of approaches to money-laundering regulation, which may be combined or remain separate. They both involve making key private-sector entrepreneurs primarily responsible for implementing public policy goals and developing (or attempting to develop) an interpenetrating private-public "security quilt." Apart from any preventive effects that they may have—which have not yet been established but which plausibly exist—such controls are useful primarily for ex post facto audit trails partly because of the sheer volume of cash transfer and suspicious activity reports, which without electronic delivery and some good analytic software programs, is too slow to be dynamically useful.

The first general approach, adopted first in the United States and then in Australia but in no other major financial centers in the world, involves routine currency transaction reporting (CTR), domestic and cross-border by specified financial intermediaries—banks, but sometimes also *bureaux de change*, casinos, and even car dealers—for any currency transaction beyond a specified threshold (generally $10,000) and identification of their customers at least at this threshold.

The second general approach, adopted throughout Europe and the major Far Eastern centers such as Hong Kong and Japan, requires or permits intermediaries to make suspicious transaction reports but not routine cash deposit reports. This system is meant to provide more discriminating and practically useful information relative to a CTR system, and the United States has gradually supplemented its CTRs with suspicious activity reports; Australia always operated the combined system (Austrac 2000; Department of Justice 2001). U.S. federal agencies proposed regulations that would require financial service providers to develop customer profiles and determine the source of funds that may be incommensurate with a customer's profile or typical banking activity. However, my interviews indicate that following widespread opposition justified on the grounds of privacy concerns and organized by an e-mail lobby of bankers (in unusual collaboration with left- and right-wing privacy enthusiasts) to Congress and the media, these proposals were withdrawn in 2000 until terrorism reoriented privacy values in 2001. In any event, the Federal Reserve Board and state departments of banking such as that in New York attempt to ensure compliance with the Bank Secrecy Act, via examination and audit functions and via dissemination of anti-money-laundering guidance procedures for regulated banks.[5] These reporting and monitoring controls are supplemented by enhanced (though largely unfunded) financial investigative efforts in designated high intensity financial crimes areas such as New York, Los

Angeles, and the U.S.-Mexico border areas.

There is a third type, more comprehensive than the second, whereby institutions are required to report unusual transactions to a civilian body, which then examines them to see if there is any reason to classify them as suspicious; if there is deemed to be such a reason, then the report is passed onto the criminal investigation authorities. The aim here is partly to protect privacy in systems prone to overdisclosure.

In an attempt to cut across the multiplicity of jurisdictional issues and reduce their regulatory costs and the serious reputational damage they were suffering in the media mostly for the money of corrupt dictators rather than for anything having to do with drugs, a number of banks agreed at Wolfsberg in 2000 to establish a common global standard for their private banking operations (i.e., for very wealthy clients only). These Wolfsberg Principles include common due diligence procedures for opening and keeping watch over accounts, especially those identified as belonging to politically exposed persons (i.e., potentially corrupt public officials) who may sometimes combine corruption with drug money laundering.

The effects of antilaundering measures

Given the political and social importance of this area, the absence of evaluation research on it and organized crime generally is remarkable. What sorts of effects might one seek to identify? These may be divided into process effects (e.g., on private and public enforcement practices) and impact effects (which require a deeper understanding of the organization of crime than we currently have and are very difficult to measure in practice), including (1) the prosecution or other incapacitation of offenders, (2) the organization of crime, and (3) levels of crime (in the context of this article, drug use and sales).

In terms of process, the world's legal landscape has been transformed in slightly more than a decade, with almost every country and territory—including almost all offshore financial centers—adopting laws permitting or requiring disclosure and mutual legal assistance, even though their conformity with the forty measures (or principles) mandated by FATF may vary. Usually following a major scandal, some countries and financial institutions have sought to become market leaders in compliance against drug money laundering, thereby intentionally creating an unlevel playing field. Territories such as the Cayman Islands (blacklisted in 2000 but delisted in 2001) or Jersey (now accepted as well regulated) attempt to persuade wealthy corporate investors to do business there.[6] Conversely, rogue jurisdictions market their privacy and asset protection trusts that are impenetrable to inquisitive countries, especially to their tax inspectors. Yet while compliance might be excellent generally (and the bank might even refuse bribes from undercover Drug Enforcement Agency agents[7]), a favored client—an influential politician and/or drug trafficker in

Colombia, Mexico, or Peru—may be given special treatment. Hence the importance of the Wolfsberg Principles as a counterweight to local temptations to service powerful clients or potential clients, whether narcokleptocrats or "merely" corrupt heads of state and their families.

Levels of visible enforcement of antilaundering provisions—prosecutions or deauthorizations of financial and professional intermediaries for money laundering or failing to institute proper measures of regulation—have been extremely modest.[8] Furthermore, those prosecuted—like BCCI and some Mexican banks after the controversial Operation Casablanca in which American agents organized a sting against Mexican banks in Mexico and the United States—or those prohibited from banking tend to be foreign or marginal banks rather than mainstream global banks whose private banking operations were particularly prone to abuse pre-Wolfsberg. There is little doubt that scandals such as that engulfing the Bank of New York over the alleged laundering of Russian mafia money have a powerful effect on refocusing the compliance function of that bank and of other banks with known Russian clients, though it is not clear how much Russian money was related, respectively, to drugs, to organized crime, or to capital flight searching for an economically and politically safer home.

As for impact on enforcement, it has been difficult to find police support for radical shifts in staff from equally prized and media-supported areas of crime and disorder to financial investigation. Many U.S. state and local forces have become highly dependant on income from federal equitable sharing and adoptive forfeiture, and there is some evidence of goal displacement as enforcement agencies target forfeitable assets rather than serious offenders (Blumenson and Nilsen 1998). This has not happened elsewhere, partly because postconviction reversal of the burden of proof typically yields modest results and, crime proceeds income is not redirected toward the police (Freiberg and Fox 2000; Levi 2001). As for impact on territories and on the private sector, following regional action plans, few high integrity/capital security places offer high secrecy any more, imposing informational uncertainties and extra costs on launderers.

In theory, suspicious transaction reporting by bankers offers the possibility of policing in a less prejudiced way than by use of police discretion, via dispassionate computer-modeled neural network analysis. However, although expensive software throws up more sophisticated methodologies to pursue, we note the same criteria of suspiciousness—of out-of-context behavior largely by "the usual suspects"—that the police use, only operated this time by bankers (Levi 1991; Gold and Levi 1994). Observation suggests that efforts made in Australia, the Netherlands, and the United Kingdom to develop good collaborative relationships with the financial sector in the early years produced greater willingness to respond positively, and efforts made by Austrac to develop good interagency relationships with law enforcement likewise produced greater acceptance of the value of their work.

Demonstrable impact on crime and even on crime detection remains harder to identify, however. Methodological problems in linking causes to effects mean that there are few defensible positive findings about the direct, short-term impact of money-laundering reporting on prosecutions and on confiscation.[9] Moreover, Indo-Pak or Chinese communities have well-established underground banking mechanisms or informal value transmission systems that predate banking and that also are relatively immune from surveillance by the police and tax authorities (see Passas 1999), though the focus on terrorist finance will put more pressure on them.

Based on an analysis of what happened to one thousand suspicious transaction reports made in the United Kingdom during the early 1990s, Gold and Levi (1994) concluded that at the (now tripled) rate of thirteen thousand disclosures a year, the entire money-laundering reporting system produced an unambiguous yield of only thirteen drug trafficking—including money laundering—convictions annually. At a time when reporting for nondrug suspicions was rarer than today, this still yielded some thirty-five more convictions for fraud and for other serious offences. There is no research equivalent for the United States, but FinCEN's (1999) annual report states that suspicious activity reports represent less than 5 percent of the thirty-five thousand or so Bank Secrecy Act reports accessed for "ongoing investigations or prosecutions" in 1999 via its Gateway terminal. Any longer-term impact in terms of building up patterns of information—however plausible—remains hypothetical in light of current knowledge. This disregards preventive and (increasingly attempted) crime-disruptive effects, which likewise remain unmeasured.

These modest verifiable results reflect the amount of resource put into the system by bankers, financial investigators, and prosecutors, as well as the legal framework that then required proof of the predicate offense.[10] Even allowing for very modest savings by lower-level drug sellers, the less than $1 billion forfeited annually in the United States from all crime is a modest proportion of total retail drug sales, with no obvious effect on the drug trade as a whole, whatever effect it might have on particular offenders or crime organizations.

Despite this lack of impact on the ongoing crime trade and the thriving crime markets, some interesting effects are discernible. English police have given examples of some offenders working harder to get back the capital confiscated, and the high profit margins mean that the opportunity cost of granting credit to "good criminals" whose assets have been taken is not as great as some enforcement officials might hope (Levi and Osofsky 1995). If financial investigators cannot find out where the assets are or who owns them, they can make it hard (and expensive) for the traffickers and launderers to collect the money, but this may not show up in their confiscation yield. Laundering costs allegedly rose from 6 to 8 percent at the beginning of the 1980s to up to 20 percent by the mid-1990s (United Nations International Drug Control Programme 1997, 141) and (according to U.S. drug law enforcement sources) substantially more today, though this does not tell us how the amount of laundering has changed, or even whether people are doing the same sort of thing but demanding more "rent" for taking heavier risks.[11] Early research results from the Netherlands show that typical offender flexibility in offence commission and money laundering may be much lower than we believe (van Duyne 1998; van Duyne and de Miranda 1999). The cost of laundering in different parts of the world and for different predicate crimes requires more research.

Particular money-laundering techniques vary by the need to launder and the skill set and contacts of particular offenders, which may change over time. One would have to follow the altered behavior (or inability to change) of the same or similar offender groups to examine the impact of antilaundering measures.[12] Despite work on money-laundering typologies by and for the FATF and other bodies such as the Council of Europe, we lack more than a modest understanding of the incidence and prevalence of current techniques even from the systematic analysis of detected cases, let alone from those that are undetected.

CONCLUSION

It is difficult to imagine now what levels of use of different drugs or the organization of crime would have looked like had money-laundering controls taken a different form or not existed at all in many countries. In a short period, an almost global compatible (if not harmonized and centrally policed) infrastructure has been created within which private-public partnerships (however tense at times) can be developed. However, despite the increasing development of intrainstitutional and governmental neural networks for sniffing out unusual or profiled behavior—Austrac conducts electronic monitoring of some 5 million international transfers a year—this new world order fights an unequal battle with the low transparency of international electronic funds transfers and their sheer volume, which overwhelms bank systems still largely based on human judgments of suspiciousness. Detected drug money laundering cases vary enormously in sophistication but typically are lower than in corporate fraud and transnational corruption cases. However skeptical one is about the proportion of income from crime that is saved—and especially the proportion of offenders who save significant amounts—the vast disparity between plausible proceeds and actual confiscations/forfeitures suggests that there must be a continuous accumulation of mutant capitalism.[13] What the effects of these funds are and where they are located remain obscure. Nor—partly due to inherent methodological difficulties—is it obvious what effects antilaundering and forfeiture policies have had on the levels of drug production, distribution, and use. The threat of international sanctions may be used against banks that handle the accounts of businesses that sell drug-related products even where they are tolerated locally (in the Netherlands, more recently in Belgium, and in Switzerland, which has never ratified the 1988 Vienna UN Convention). We thus see how the integrated global financial system, combined with a money-laundering focus, pressurizes conformity and economic exclusion for alternative models of dealing with drug problems. It can always be argued that following the money simply needs to be pursued more rigorously with more resources in more countries, but even those unpersuaded by Naylor's (1999) vigorous critique might keep an open mind on the effectiveness of antilaundering and forfeiture policies for reducing levels of drug supplies, whatever effects such a focus might have on reducing harm from corruption, fraud, and major crime proceeds as a whole.

Notes

1. However, Australia, Belgium, Germany, and the Netherlands, for example, had very broad coverage of predicate crimes right from the beginning.

2. Laundering charges tend to produce evil empire images in the popular mind. I am not suggesting that this prioritization of drug trafficking over fraud is appropriate; this is a sociological judgment about the populist and media-fuelled value hierarchies in many contemporary societies.

3. Thus far, there appears to be no such qualitative research on the nature of money laundering prosecutions. Relatively trivial events can be used for tactical reasons against major offenders simply because they are the most serious offences with demonstrable connections to the targets. Al Capone's conviction for tax evasion was merely one early example, but where organized crime groups are involved in multiple offense types, such flexibility of prosecutions is to be expected.

4. Banks may have corporate criminal liability in the United States if it is concluded that any bank official knew that he or she was structuring a series of transactions below the $10,000 reporting threshold.

5. As in other areas of drug enforcement, overlapping agency mandates generate rivalry between regulators.

6. I have chosen these jurisdictions because they both suffered serious reputational damage for drug and fraud scandals in the past.

7. We may hear about institutions that do take bribes in undercover sting operations, but no details are available about those who do not, leading to a perceptual imbalance in judgments about how corruption-prone institutions are. Even the Miami branch of Bank of Credit and Commerce International (BCCI) initially refused requests of undercover operatives to launder money for them.

8. Proposals in the draft Second European Union Directive 2000 to require lawyers to report suspected money laundering by their clients, passed in the aftermath of 9/11, aroused tremendous opposition. In the United Kingdom, lawyers have been included since 1986, though the number of suspicious transactions they report remains very low. In the United Kingdom, strong efforts were made from the start to involve all financial and professional bodies cooperatively.

9. At the risk of being fatuous, this means neither that there is an impact nor that there is no impact.

10. On the other hand, nor is there evidence yet of the impact that larger investments in financial investigation can have. Such investigation can have broader usefulness in assisting crime investigation.

11. To the extent that offenders are well informed, how do we find out about the extent of what they have done, except where the flows are so gross—for instance, the flows of money into Austrian banks from Indonesia in the first quarter of 1998—that they cannot be accounted for except arguably as illegal capital flight?

12. Interviews and intelligence from the United Kingdom suggest that larger volumes of cash are having to be stored since placement within the United Kingdom has become more difficult.

13. In the felicitous phrase of Sir David Omand, former permanent secretary to the British Home Office.

References

Austrac. 2000. *Annual report 2000*. Canberra: Commonwealth of Australia.

Blum, Jack, Michael Levi, R. Tom Naylor, and Phil Williams. 1998. *Financial havens, banking secrecy and money-laundering*. Issue 8 of *UNDCP technical series*. New York: United Nations.

Blumenson, Eric, and Eva Nilsen. 1998. Policing for profit: The drug war's hidden economic agenda. *University of Chicago Law Review* 65:35-114.

de Soto, Hernando. 2000. *The mystery of capital*. New York: Bantam.

Department of Justice. 2001. *The SAR activity review 2: Trends, tips & issues*. Washington DC: Bank Secrecy Act Advisory Group.

FinCEN. 1999. *FINCEN follows the money*. Washington, DC: U.S. Department of the Treasury.

Freiberg, Arie, and Richard Fox. 2000. Evaluating the effectiveness of Australia's confiscation laws. *Australian and New Zealand Journal of Criminology* 33 (3): 239-65.

Gilmore, William. 1999. *Dirty money: The evolution of money-laundering counter-measures*. Amsterdam: Council of Europe Press.

Gold, Michael, and Michael Levi. 1994. *Money-laundering in the UK: An appraisal of suspicion-based reporting*. London: Police Foundation.

Levi, Michael. 1991. Pecunia non olet: Cleansing the money launderers from the temple. *Crime, Law, & Social Change* 16:217-302.

———. 1997. Evaluating the "new policing": Attacking the money trail of organised crime. *Australian and New Zealand Journal of Criminology* 30:1-25.

———. 2001. *Best practice report no. 3: Reversal of the burden of proof in confiscation of the proceeds of crime*. Strasbourg, France: Council of Europe.

Levi, Michael, and Lisa Osofsky. 1995. *Investigating, seizing, and confiscating the proceeds of crime*. Crime Detection and Prevention Series paper no. 61. London: Home Office.

Maguire, Mike. 2000. Policing by risks and targets: Some dimensions and implications of intelligence-led crime control. *Policing and Society* 9:1-22.

Naylor, R. Tom. 1999. *Follow-the-money methods in crime control policy*. Toronto, Canada: Nathanson Centre for the Study of Organized Crime and Corruption.

Office of National Drug Control Strategy. 2001. *The national drug control strategy: 2001*. Annual report. Washington, DC: Government Printing Office.

Passas, Nikos. 1999. *Informal value transfer systems and criminal organizations: A study into so-called underground banking networks*. The Hague, the Netherlands: Dutch Ministry of Justice, Onderzoeksnotities.

Reuter, Peter. 2000. Assessing alternative methodologies for estimating revenues from illicit drugs. Unpublished manuscript.

Stessens, Guy. 2000. Money laundering: An international enforcement model. Cambridge, UK: Cambridge University Press.

United Nations International Drug Control Programme. 1997. *World drug report*. Oxford, UK: Oxford University Press.

van Duyne, Petrus C. 1998. Money-laundering: Pavlov's dog and beyond. *Howard Journal of Criminal Justice* 37 (4): 359-74.

van Duyne, Petrus C., and Hervey de Miranda. 1999. The emperor's clothes of disclosure: Hot money and suspect disclosures. *Crime, Law and Social Change* 3:245-71.

Walker, J. 1999. *A logical approach to the quantification of global money laundering from the international illicit drugs trade*. Canberra: Commonwealth of Australia.

REVIEW ARTICLE

Black Flower: Prisons and the Future of Incarceration

HALLINAN, JOSEPH T. 2001. *Going up the River: Travels in a Prison Nation*. New York: Random House.

LIN, ANN CHIH. 2000. *Reform in the Making: The Implementation of Social Policy in Prison*. Princeton, NJ: Princeton University Press.

TONRY, MICHAEL, and RICHARD S. FRASE, eds. 2001. *Sentencing and Sanctions in Western Countries*. Oxford, UK: Oxford University Press.

TONRY, MICHAEL, and JOAN PETERSILIA, eds. 1999. *Prisons: Crime and Justice—A Review of Research*. Vol. 26. Chicago: University of Chicago Press.

ZIMRING, FRANKLIN E., GORDON HAWKINS, and SAM KAMIN. 2001. *Punishment and Democracy: Three Strikes and You're Out in California*. Oxford, UK: Oxford University Press.

Marie Gottschalk is an assistant professor in the Department of Political Science at the University of Pennsylvania. She is the author of The Shadow Welfare State: Business, Labor, and Health Policy in the United States *(2000, Cornell University Press). A former editor and journalist, she was a visiting scholar in 2001-2002 at the Russell Sage Foundation. She is currently working on a book about the politics of mass incarceration in the United States.*

NOTE: I would like to thank Mary Fainsod Katzenstein of Cornell University for her helpful comments on an earlier draft. I am indebted to Eric Lomazoff and Sabina Neem for their invaluable research assistance and to the Russell Sage Foundation for supporting this project.

Almost two centuries ago, Nathaniel Hawthorne (cited in Christianson 1998) suggested that prison is a necessary but not entirely desirable social institution, describing it as "the black flower of our civilization" (p. 312). He implied that prisons were durable weeds that refused to die. During the past three decades, this black flower has proliferated in the United States as the country has embarked on a prison-building boom without precedent here or elsewhere. In a period dominated by calls to roll back the state in all areas of social and economic policy, we have witnessed a massive expansion of the state in the area of penal policy.

Unlike other major state-building exercises like the New Deal and the Great Society, the new penal policy was not presented as a package for public debate. It emerged rapidly during the past thirty years largely outside of the public eye and was not necessarily planned out. While the explosion in the size of the prison population is well documented, the underlying causes and consequences of this massive expansion and the possibilities for reversing it are not well understood. And what understanding there is has not helped to fundamentally shift penal policies in a more constructive direction. The five works discussed here are critical contributions to understanding the causes, consequences, and dynamics of the boom in the prison population. While their central focus is not how to reform U.S. penal policies, these analyses do have important public policy implications for anyone interested in how to reduce the country's incarceration rate.

In reviewing these books, I develop several interrelated themes. First, I catalogue the various causal arguments that these authors propose to explain the rapid growth of incarceration in the United States. These include changes in the political culture, an increase in drug-related crimes, and economic arguments about who benefits from mass incarceration. Taken alone or together, these arguments do not completely or satisfactorily explain American exceptionalism in penal policy. Second, I suggest that the problem needs to be viewed in a comparative perspective. Comparing the penal policies and institutions of the United States with those of other advanced industrialized countries and examining significant variations across the fifty states illuminate the underlying causes. The specific institutional context of American politics helps explain the ready politicization of crime as an issue. Politicization of crime, in turn, has driven up rates of incarceration. The most notable example of this among these works is the case of California. Finally, I discuss the pressing public policy issue of how the high rates of incarceration might be reversed. I argue that the right question to ask in this context is not whether the political elite, the public, or the criminal experts hold the key to unlock the prison doors. In the longer run, we must ask, Under what conditions can an anti-mass-incarceration coalition of political leaders, the public, and the experts be crafted? These five works taken together suggest the need for such an alliance.

CAUSES OF THE BOOM

From the mid-1920s to the early 1970s, the incarceration rate in the United States was remarkably stable, averaging 110 state and federal prisoners per 100,000 people (Blumstein and Beck 1999, 17).[1] While the U.S. rate tended to be higher, it did not radically exceed the incarceration rates of other advanced industrialized countries. Since the early 1970s, the U.S. rate of imprisonment has accelerated dramatically, resulting in a fivefold increase in the incarcerated population between 1973 and 1997 (Caplow and Simon 1999, 63). Today, the rate of incarceration in prison is 478 per 100,000. If jailed inmates are included, the rate jumps to 699 per 100,000, which is six to ten times the rate of the Western European countries (Beck and Harrison 2001, Table 1:2, Table 3:3; Tonry 2001, 9).[2] This constitutes a higher proportion of the adult population than any other country in the world except Russia (Currie 1998, 15). The United States, with 5 percent of the world's population, has 25 percent of its prisoners (Gonnerman 2000, 56). Even after taking into account important qualifications in use of the standard 100,000 yardstick to compare incarceration rates cross-nationally, the United States remains off the charts.[3]

These overall figures on incarceration belie the enormous and disproportionate impact that mass imprisonment has had on certain groups in U.S. society. Since 1980, the proportion of inmates who are African American has increased sharply.

Blacks, who make up less than 13 percent of the U.S. population, now comprise more than half of all prison inmates, up from one-third twenty years ago and one-quarter in the late 1930s (Tonry 1995, 29; Jaynes and Williams, cited in Friedman 1993, 378). By the mid-1990s, the combined incarceration (prison and jail) rate for adult black males in the United States was nearly 7,000 per 100,000 compared to about 900 per 100,000 for adult white males (Bureau of Justice Statistics, Table 6.12, cited in Reitz 2001, 244). The population of women in U.S. prisons has risen more than eightfold during the past two decades. During that time, the average annual growth of the number of women behind bars has well exceeded that of male prisoners (Chesney-Lind 1998, 66; Beck and Harrison 2001, Table 7; Talvi 2001, 1). The absolute number of women in prison in the United States is larger than the entire prison populations of France, Germany, or England (Tonry and Petersilia 1999, 10; Pollock-Byrne 1990).

The impact of the rising prison and jail population extends far beyond the 2 million men and women who are currently incarcerated in the United States. On any given day, more than 5 million people are under the supervision of the correctional system, including parole, probation, and other community supervision sanctions. This constitutes nearly 3 percent of the total resident population, a rate of state supervision that is unprecedented in U.S. history (Bureau of Justice Statistics, cited in Caplow and Simon 1999, 73). If one adds up the total number of inmates, parolees, probationers, employees of correctional institutions, close relatives of inmates and correctional employees, and residents in communities where jails and prisons are major employers, tens of millions of people are directly affected each year by prisons and jails (Tonry and Petersilia 1999, vii).

What accounts for this unprecedented change in U.S. incarceration rates? Criminal justice experts, with some notable exceptions, generally agree that "changes in penal policies and practices, not changes in crime rates" are the primary explanation, "but there is disagreement about the cause of penal policy changes" (Caplow and Simon 1999, 63). Experts identify a range of causes for these changes in penal policies, including shifts in U.S. political culture, the role of criminal justice experts, the expanding trade in illegal drugs, and the underlying structure of American politics. Many activists in the burgeoning movement against mass incarceration stress the enormous and growing political clout of the multi-billion-dollar corrections industry. How valid are these respective explanations?

Penal populism. Franklin E. Zimring, Gordon Hawkins, and Sam Kamin contended that populism is driving this expansion. The populism that they described in *Punishment and Democracy*, a compelling account of the 1994 enactment and subsequent implementation of California's "three strikes and you're out" legislation, operates in subtle ways. It is not merely an extension of the law-and-order politics that burst onto the national stage with Barry Goldwater's 1964 campaign and has been a prominent feature of subsequent presidential, state, and local electoral contests, most notoriously in George H. W. Bush's 1988 demonization of Willie Horton. In their view, the social authority accorded criminal justice experts in the late nineteenth century and first half of the twentieth century "prevented the direct domination of policy by antioffender sentiments that are consistently held by most citizens most of the time" (p. 15). This helped to prevent a massive expansion of the penal state despite growing public unease about crime and the social dislocations caused by rapid industrialization and urbanization. In more recent years, politicians and the public have locked the experts out of the policymaking process, thus permitting penal populism to flourish.

Zimring, Hawkins, and Kamin attributed the nation's increasingly punitive stance and the related sidelining of the experts to the widespread phenomenon of growing mistrust in government. As citizen mistrust of government has grown, the public desires to limit the discretion of state officials to perform all sorts of activities, from collecting and spending taxes to deciding what happens to those who break the law. California's 1976 Determinate Sentencing Law, which essentially eliminated parole by curtailing the parole board's authority to determine release dates, is a prime example of this, as is Proposition 13, the ballot initiative to slash property taxes in the golden state that propelled the tax revolt of the 1970s. *Punishment and Democracy* portrayed California's three strikes measure, which established the use of tough, mandatory sentences after second and third convictions for certain felonies, in a similar light because it greatly restricts the discretion of California judges. "At its core, then, Three Strikes represents a jurisprudence of mistrust rather than any particular theory of punishment," (p. 174) they argued.

Punishment and Democracy attempts to explain two tantalizing paradoxes in penal policy. First, the more that citizens doubt the government's capacity to solve problems, the greater their willingness to invest in prisons, which, after all, are costly state structures. "Soaring prison populations are a manifestation of mistrust in government because the unwillingness to delegate power in individual cases makes attempts to increase punishments in the system depend on blunt instruments" (p. 175) like prisons, the authors explained. The second paradox is that the enormous rise in violent crime from 1964 to 1974 had surprisingly little effect on legislation or the administration of criminal justice. By contrast, penal policies became increasingly punitive in the early 1990s in the face of falling crime rates. Zimring, Hawkins, and Kamin speculated that the absence of a consensus in the late 1960s and early 1970s about what government could do to reduce crime might explain the relatively low levels of government involvement during that period. Sustained declines in crime in the 1990s fueled public confidence about the ability of public authorities

to make streets safer. "The effort to pass laws can more easily be justified when citizens believe that legal change can generate palpable improvement in crime rates" (p. 165), the authors explained.

Weakness of the state. Crime now occupies a prominent place in U.S. political culture in a way it did not previously for several reasons, according to Theodore Caplow and Jonathan Simon (1999). The first is the relative weakness of the state. Echoing Zimring and his coauthors, they suggested that declining public confidence in social welfare programs and state interventions in the national economy are evidence of that weakness, as are periodic surges in the crime rate that have "diminished the prestige of governments in their most traditional function of maintaining civil order" (p. 79). The decline in public confidence in social welfare programs has removed an important set of tools that the state could once use to tackle pressing social problems. Intensification of crime-control activities is an attractive way for the state to burnish the image of its competence and restore its sense of purpose. "Punishment invokes a primordial understanding of state power that remains highly credible. Imprisonment, especially when promoted as incapacitation, is something government knows it can accomplish," Caplow and Simon (1999, 79-80) explained. Thus, the "politics of punishment" are no longer subordinated to the "politics of welfare" (Caplow and Simon 1999, 70-71). This echoes a central theme of David Garland's earlier work and his new book *The Culture of Control* (2001).

Caplow and Simon (1999), like Garland (2001) in his admittedly broad-brush book, do not present detailed, careful analyses of public opinion data to document this supposed fundamental shift in public opinion. They are on strong ground when they claim that public confidence in the government is declining, as evidenced by responses over the years to standard survey questions such as, "How much of the time do you trust the government in Washington to do the right thing?" (Caplow and Simon 1999, 80).[4] They are less convincing, however, when they claim that this drop in trust has resulted in a wholesale rejection of public social programs, excepting a few sacred cows like social security, resulting in a delegitimization of the state and a need for government officials to regain their legitimacy by promoting harsher penal policies. This important connection is not well demonstrated. Indeed, they cite one study showing the contrary, namely, that the basic political orientation of Americans (where citizens locate themselves on the liberal-conservative continuum) has shifted much less over the years than many assume (Caplow and Simon 1999, 69). This is consistent with recent public opinion data indicating widespread public support for a range of government interventions from education to health care to protecting the environment (Berke and Elder 2001, A-1; Harwood and Cummings 2001, A-18).

The role of public opinion in penal policy is extremely complex. For all the talk about a more punitive public mood, the public's anxiety about crime is "subject to sudden, dramatic shifts, unrelated to any objective measure of crime" (Frase 2001, 268).[5] Elsewhere in their chapter, Caplow and Simon (1999) appeared to take a more nuanced view of public opinion. What in fact may be taking place is not so much a fundamental shift in U.S. public opinion about social welfare programs and so forth but a widening gap between elite and mass opinion. Political elites are more willing now to play the crime card to harvest votes because of important changes in the structure of U.S. politics.[6] These shifts in elite opinion and strategy, in turn, may have such profound effects on penal policy because of the particular institutional context of the United States overall, and of certain states in particular, notably California, a point I will come back to.

The crucial factor may not be that the center of public opinion has moved to the right as Americans have turned away from the welfare state. Rather, there may no longer be any real center that dominates U.S. politics. As a result, "today's center is little more than a floating set of preferences on a vast range of issues, charted by polls and pundits," Caplow and Simon (1999, 81) suggested. With the rise of new social movements in the United States and other postindustrial societies, the new politics of values and identity have replaced or submerged the more traditional conflicts over wealth and national security, they contended. When the center is fluid and up for grabs, the victim-offender fault line becomes a much more significant demarcation in politics. Being for victims and against offenders is a simple equation that can help knit together politically disparate groups ranging from the more traditional, conservative, law-and-order constituencies mobilized around punitive policies like three strikes; to feminist movements organized against rape and domestic violence; to gay and lesbian groups advocating for hate crimes legislation; to the million moms pushing for gun control.[7] "If the postmaterialist politics tends toward issues of good and evil, crime is a natural metaphor for evil" Caplow and Simon (p. 84) suggested. Zimring, Hawkins, and Kamin echoed this view when they argued that punishment policy has become a "zero-sum competition" between crime victims (good) and criminal offenders (evil). Citizens no longer have to calculate costs and benefits of various policies. All they have to do is choose sides. Since the "implicit assumption is that anything that is bad for offenders must be beneficial to victims" (Zimring, Hawkins, and Kamin 2001, 223), the offenders lose out every time.

The new drug trade. Changes in the political culture alone do not explain why demands for punitive justice have become unprecedented in their intensity. Earlier periods of public alarm over crime, notably during Prohibition in the late 1920s and again in the late 1930s, resulted in far more modest increases in incarceration rates. And contrary to the pattern of the past thirty years, incarceration rates did not continue to

climb steadily higher but were cyclical. They retreated after peaking in 1931 and then again in 1939. "For political mobilization around law and order to produce a sustained increase in imprisonment, other conditions must be present," according to Caplow and Simon (1999, 93). One important condition is the availability of a large pool of offenders to be imprisoned. They argued that important changes in the drug trade coupled with the get-tough stance on drugs declared by Presidents Ronald Reagan and George H. W. Bush provided that opening.

Both the number and the proportion of drug offenders in prison have exploded. In 1980, the drug incarceration rate was 15 inmates in state and federal prisons per 100,000 adults. By 1996, the rate had increased more than ninefold to 148 per 100,000, "a rate greater than that for the entire U.S. prison system in the fifty years to 1973" (Blumstein and Beck 1999, 20-21). By contrast, the percentage of people sentenced to U.S. prisons for violent crimes is relatively low (29.5 percent in 1996) and has not increased since 1991 (Bureau of Justice Statistics, Table 1.23, cited in Tonry 2001, 14).

The scale of drug enterprises expanded rapidly in the 1980s with the introduction of new drugs and distribution strategies, most notably for crack cocaine, according to Caplow and Simon (1999). They suggested that the rise of a large retail drug sales force furnished a nearly unlimited pool of offenders. Here they may be overstating the degree to which changes in the structure of the drug trade independently fed the politics of mass incarceration. There is always a potentially unlimited pool of offenders available because "deviance is not a property *inherent* in any particular kind of behavior" (Erikson 1966, 6). Rather, deviance is a property conferred on a certain behavior by the majority or by the powerful. Crime waves or moral panics, such as the war on drugs, do not necessarily entail increases in the volume of deviance. They do involve "a rash of publicity, a moment of excitement and alarm, a feeling that something needs to be done" (Erikson 1966, 69).[8] Despite all the bluster, the volume of deviants who come to a community's attention is likely to remain fairly constant because there are finite limits to a community's capacity to detect and punish deviance (Erikson 1966, 163). What is exceptional in the U.S. case is that those limits appear to have been broken during the past three decades. The moral panics over crime and drugs are no longer just symbolic politics with few lasting and concrete consequences.

The history of drug policy from the Nixon years onward is a good case in point. The Nixon administration and the U.S. Congress initially treated marijuana and casual drug use as benign deviances not worthy of serious punishment. Despite Nixon's stress on law-and-order themes in the 1968 presidential campaign, rates of imprisonment fell during his first term in office. In 1970, leaders of both parties applauded when Congress eliminated almost all federal mandatory minimum sentences for drug offenders.[9] The Nixon administration subsequently shifted the emphasis of its drug policy from treatment of hard-core users to punishment for both casual users and addicts. It did so to protect its right flank after New York Governor Nelson Rockefeller declared that addiction had become a plague that threatened the lives of innocent middle-class children and in 1973 pushed through his draconian drug laws.[10] Nixon's new drug policy also provided a convenient cover to reorganize various agencies of the government to better serve the electoral and perceived national security needs of his administration (Epstein 1977, 53). Reagan and Bush subsequently declared a war on drugs because it served similar needs and because of the emergence in the late 1970s of a powerful grassroots movement of suburban parents bent on shifting the terms of the debate about drugs from public health to morality, fueling the zero tolerance stance that has undergirded drug policy for so many years (Massing 1998, chap. 11).

U.S. incarceration rates began their upward climb at the start of the second term of the Nixon administration, years before Reagan and Bush enlisted the country for an all-out war on drugs. They continued to climb steadily during the 1970s, even though the country appeared ready to decriminalize marijuana on the eve of the 1976 election and even though the Carter administration took a more tolerant attitude toward drug use (Massing 1998, 137). Reagan and Bush declared a war on drugs and pushed for tougher penalties for drug offenders in the 1980s despite evidence of continually falling drug use.[11] All of this gives one pause in concluding that the appearance of crack cocaine and other changes in the dynamics of the drug trade conveniently furnished an unlimited supply of offenders who had previously been unavailable and thus were a major reason behind the exploding incarceration rate.

Prison industrial complex. In *Going up the River*, Joseph T. Hallinan, a journalist specializing in criminal justice issues, provided some poignant examples of a war against drugs gone awry. In explaining the roots of the nation's prison-building boom, he emphasized how economic factors are molding penal politics and practices, including drug policy. Hallinan acknowledged that people are not being imprisoned just to make a buck but indicated that financial considerations are paramount. He attributed the race to incarcerate to the emergence of powerful private groups, such as the Corrections Corporation of America (CCA), which stand to make enormous profits from prisons, and to local communities, many of them in rural areas, that have latched onto prisons as a way to perk up their depressed economies. In attempting to explain the deeper roots of the prison-building boom, he made some questionable claims. For example, at one point he said that the federal courts set it all in motion by declaring prison overcrowding and other penal conditions unconstitutional. This, in his view, forced states to make costly improvements and to subject their penal policies to market forces (p. 30).

Hallinan provided numerous colorful examples of the wide range of individuals and corporations

profiting handsomely from the burgeoning corrections industry. AT&T has its eye on the estimated $1 billion in phone calls that inmates place each year. In Tamms, Illinois, citizens so loved their new supermax prison, which cost $120,000 per cell to build, that a local sandwich shop renamed its specialty in honor of the prison: the supermax burger. Like the prison, Hallinan was told, it came with the works. The stock for the CCA, the country's oldest and largest prison company, soared more than 1,000 percent after its inception in 1983 (Hallinan 2001, xiv-xv, xvi, 125).[12] In Wallens Ridge, Virginia, the electronically armed fence that surrounds the new $77.5 million prison is a source of pride for prison officials. It is identical to the sophisticated sixteen-foot-high fence used by the Israeli government on the Golan Heights, according to the warden (p. 204). Hallinan portrayed the annual convention of the American Correctional Association, the largest private correctional organization in the country and once the epicenter of prison reform activities in the United States, as largely a corporate-sponsored trade fair for penal gadgets and services (p. 156).

Warden after warden told Hallinan that running a prison today is like running a business. Prison administrators now do time in the public sector, then cash in on their experience and connections to become "prison millionaires" at private firms servicing or operating prisons. *Going up the River* shows how the revolving door between the public and private sectors and the increased pressure to run prisons like businesses have fueled corruption and distorted public priorities. At a minimum, this revolving door has created potential conflicts of interest. Michael Quinlan, the former head of the Federal Bureau of Prisons, retired in 1992 and became chief executive of a spin-off company of the CCA. Edwin Meese III, Reagan's attorney general, is chairman of the Enterprise Prison Institute, a group pushing to make inmate labor more accessible to private industry. Morgan Reynolds, another enthusiast of prison labor, told Hallinan that prison administrators in the past had been blind to the commercial potential of their institutions. But now, those opportunities hold the key to their success. "It's pretty clear," he explained to Hallinan, "that's where the future is if we're going to grow our prison population" (p. 173-74, 148).

While Hallinan included numerous testimonies by enthusiastic prison administrators, staff, and members of the community, he provided little hard evidence about how prisons have actually buoyed local economies. Some activists involved in the burgeoning movement against mass incarceration are taking aim at what they claim is a myth that prisons constitute a critical public works program for economically distressed communities. Ruth Wilson Gilmore, a professor of geography at the University of California, Berkeley, who is working on a book about prisons in California, has compared the economies of counties with and without prisons. All things being equal, counties without prisons did better economically than counties with them

(Ruth Wilson Gilmore 2001). Craig Gilmore, who assists residents in rural California to organize against building more prisons, says that local communities are often suckered into becoming boosters for a prison and that the purported economic windfall does not materialize (Craig Gilmore 2001).[13] Hallinan's account of Youngstown, Ohio's deep disillusionment after the CCA built a brand new prison there bolsters this view. "Knowing what I know now," said the disappointed mayor of Youngstown, "I would never have allowed CCA to build a prison here" (p. 185).

Hallinan himself stressed that the more money spent on prisons means less money available for other public services. This has become an important rallying point for many prison reform activists, who emphasize the trade-off between funding for prisons and funding for education in particular. In New York State between 1988 and 1998, spending on prisons soared $761.3 million while state allocations for state and city colleges plummeted by $615 million—almost an exact dollar-for-dollar trade-off (Gangi, Schiraldi, and Ziedenberg, cited in Hallinan 2001, 104-105). California spends more on its prisons than on its two premier university systems, the University of California and California State University (p. 105).

Many activists seeking to reverse the nation's penal policies echo Hallinan's view that the emergence of a powerful prison industrial complex is the main engine driving the nation's prison-building boom.[14] While *Going up the River* provides lots of ammunition for this position, there are several problems with primarily economic explanations. First, for-profit prisons are a relatively new phenomenon. The first private prison opened in 1983, a full decade into the current prison expansion. For all the talk of privatization, by the mid-1990s, there were only about 100 privately run jails and prisons in the United States holding 37,000 inmates, or a minuscule 2 percent of the country's incarcerated population.

It may well be that the dynamics driving the prison-building boom of the past thirty years are not a unitary phenomena, and thus no single explanation will suffice. In some of his other work, Zimring (2000, 2001) suggested that the period be broken up into three separate eras characterized by different politics and policies. The first phase, lasting from 1973 to the mid-1980s, involved a general increase in commitments of marginal felons. In this phase, the average sentence did not lengthen much, and no specific group of offenders was targeted. During the second phase, which he dated from the mid-1980s to the early 1990s, drug offenders were the main target as defendants convicted of drug-related crimes composed a significant proportion of the prison population for the first time. In the third phase, from the early 1990s to the present, the country has pursued harsher penalties in the face of falling crime rates. In the earlier phases, the new laws generally barked louder than they bit. In the 1990s, there was a closer linkage between the symbolic politics of being tough on criminals and the substantive policies behind the tough talk. In the current phase,

vested financial interests like private prison companies and prison guard unions may be more critical in explaining the growth of the incarcerated population than in the previous two eras.

COMPARATIVE POLITICS
OF SENTENCING AND
INCARCERATION

Powerful vested private interests, the drug trade, stresses on the welfare state, the emergence of new social movements, and penal populism are not political developments unique to the United States. Other advanced industrialized countries have faced challenges similar in kind, if not always degree. The difference is that these political developments have coincided with massive increases in the number of people behind bars in the United States, but not elsewhere. In the U.S. case, these new political developments have combined with the existing institutions and interest groups to produce a combustible mix. Whereas incarceration rates have held steady or inched up elsewhere (or in some cases, notably Finland, declined dramatically), they have skyrocketed in the United States.

Currently, there is a dearth of comparative work on criminal justice politics and policy. A new and important contribution to this slim field is *Sentencing and Sanctions in Western Countries*, edited by Michael Tonry and Richard S. Frase. This volume does an excellent job of describing and contrasting differences in sentencing practices and incarceration rates across a range of countries, including Australia, Britain, Finland, Germany, the Netherlands, and the United States. It is less useful in explaining the roots of these differences.

What is striking is that for much of the twentieth century, U.S. incarceration rates were not that exceptional. It is only within the past thirty years or so that the country has become such an anomaly. For much of the late nineteenth and twentieth centuries, the United States was incarcerating its people at rates that were generally higher, but not remarkably higher, than other Western countries. Moreover, since the late eighteenth century, most Western countries, including the United States, have experienced similar evolutions in penal theories and, in response, adopted similar penal practices consistent with whatever was the latest theory (Frase 2001, 259). That is no longer true today. Different principles now undergird the criminal justice system in the United States. In the face of the new political developments discussed above, the specific institutional and political context of the United States has provided fertile soil for certain principles to take root and not others. It remains an open question whether the principles that dominate the U.S. system are beginning to take root elsewhere and whether other countries will join the race to incarcerate.

Guiding principles. Proportionality—the idea that the punishment should be proportional to the crime committed—remains a cornerstone of the criminal justice system in many other Western countries, but not the United States. So does the principle of parsimony, which is a "principle of self-restraint" whereby milder punishments are imposed so as to reduce the extent to which the offender's life is disrupted. It is based on the belief that defendants do not forfeit their membership in the legal and moral community on conviction, nor is society absolved of its obligation to ensure the dignity and welfare of those serving time (von Hirsch 2001, 406). Another cardinal principle of many other Western systems is that no one should be punished for an offense he or she was not found guilty of. This contrasts with a cornerstone of the federal U.S. sentencing guidelines. Promulgated in 1987, the guidelines require judges not only to sentence based on what the defendant pleaded guilty to or was convicted of but to consider more serious charges that may have been withdrawn or that resulted in an acquittal.[15]

While analysts may disagree about what are the guiding principles of U.S. sentencing practices today, they do generally agree that proportionality and parsimony are not central concerns. Some contend that a new penology now competes with older strategies to be the dominant rationale for U.S. penal policies. Under the new penology, criminal justice systems have abandoned traditional concerns like rehabilitation and crime control and now are focused on how to manage a large, persistent population of offenders (Feeley and Simon 1992). Others argue that retribution, deterrence, and incapacitation, or some combination thereof, provide the dominant rationale (see, e.g., Zimring and Hawkins 1995; Rutherford 1986, 9). Retribution means punishment for wrongdoing, pure and simple. It is rooted in the belief that the guilty must pay a penalty for their crimes. Deterrence is the idea that the promise of swift, certain, and serious punishment reduces crimes by persuading offenders not to violate the law. Incapacitation is the premise that the main purpose of prison is to punish and keep offenders off the streets. While society may not be able to control what offenders do after they are released, offenders cannot harm society while they are confined or under close supervision. Thus, the "gains from merely incapacitating convicted criminals may be very large," according to James Q. Wilson (1975, 173).[16] Since Wilson popularized the idea of incapacitation more than twenty-five years ago, analysts using a variety of methodologies have found that the deterrent and incapacitative effects of incarceration in bringing down the crime rate are small and that the offenses avoided through increased incarceration have been nonviolent rather than violent crimes (Reitz 2001, 238; Currie 1985, chap. 3). *Punishment and Democracy's* careful study of the California case supports these conclusions. "The most obvious practical finding of this study is the tiny maximum impact of the new law on crime in California" (p. 105), the authors concluded.

Some experts suggest that no theory at all guides U.S. criminal justice policy today. With the decline in the 1970s of the rehabilitative ideal,[17] the U.S. criminal justice system "has lacked even the illusory clarity of a widely voiced justification" for incapacitating "as many offenders as the system can accommodate, for as long as possible," according to Kevin R. Reitz (2001, 238). If there is any operating theory at all, it is "one of collapsing distinctions among categories of criminal offenders," as more low-level offenders are treated as hardened criminals who deserve to have the book thrown at them (Reitz 2001, 240). *Punishment and Democracy* bolsters this contention. In the early days of California's three strikes law, more twenty-five years-to-life sentences were handed down as the result of a third strike for marijuana possession than for murder, rape, and kidnapping combined. In California, a trivial felony by a twice-convicted burglar will result in a longer sentence for this three-time loser than what is meted out to a nonaggravated second-degree murderer without any qualifying strikes on his or her record (Zimring, Hawkins, and Kamin 2001, 9).

Differences in institutions. With varied success, other Western countries have been better able than the United States thus far to resist mounting pressures to abandon the guiding principles of proportionality and parsimony. While the particulars may vary from country to country, a central factor appears to be differences in the institutional arrangements and the professional norms of criminal justice administrators and the judiciary. In other countries, judges and administrators are more insulated from the politicians and public opinion. While judicial autonomy has been under assault in the United States, judges elsewhere retain enormous discretion. The most extreme example is the Netherlands, where the statutory minimum term of imprisonment is one day and applies to all crimes regardless of the seriousness of the offense (Tak 2001, 172).

The roots of this insulation and the related preservation of judicial discretion vary from country to country. In Australia, judges have been more successful at retaining their autonomy compared to U.S. judges because Australian criminology and sentencing emerged "out of a legal, rather than sociological, framework" (Freiberg 2001, 35). As a result, Australia's lawyers and judiciary have dominated various government commissions and inquiries into law reform, crime, and punishment (Freiberg 2001). In England, prominent judges were involved during the past decade in some fierce public struggles as government ministers and Parliament sought to stake out a tough law-and-order position and restrict judicial discretion through measures like mandatory minimums. Judicial opposition forced Parliament to ultimately make some concessions to the judiciary's concerns about its new tough stance (Ashworth 2001, 62-91). By contrast, the U.S. judiciary has been largely a bystander in some of the major recent overhauls of the criminal justice system. Federal judges were passive witnesses to the legislative process leading up to the creation of the U.S. Sentencing Commission in 1984 and were not even able to persuade legislators to assign judges the leading role in developing the sentencing guidelines. The Judicial Conference of the United States, the governing organization of the federal judiciary, is a "cumbersome body" that has little law-making authority and is not suited for policy innovation or political lobbying (Stith and Koh 1993, 251-52). Many of the national legal associations in the United States, such as the American Bar Association, which had been actively involved in the issue of sentencing reform in the 1970s, fell silent in the 1980s and only began to enter the fray again in the 1990s (Reitz 2001, 232).

In Germany, the incarceration rate and most of the basic features of sentencing policy have remained largely unchanged for more than three decades. Differences in the institutionalization of political and legal decision making between the United States and Germany explain the relative stability of Germany's criminal justice policies. The German incarceration rate of 90 per 100,000 is less than one-sixth the U.S. rate (Tonry 2001, 9, Table 1.1). In Germany, public opinion on criminal justice and crime is more stable because of the presence of neocorporatist organizations, a disciplined party system, publicly organized news media, and the absence of extensive public opinion polling. Criminal justice policy there is generally the product of bargaining within a relatively insulated set of government actors and thus is less vulnerable to swings in public opinion and media hype over sensational crimes. Unlike U.S. officials, who bounce back and forth between the public and private sectors and academia, criminal justice administrators in Germany are career civil servants. The views of U.S. administrators

on policy issues are more influenced by loyalty to the current administrative leadership or to outside institutions, law firms, and academic or business institutions to which they may return than to political parties and the political bureaucracy, as in the German case. (Savelsberg 1994, 931-32)

The judicial appointment process is far less politicized in Germany because judges "are appointed as civil servants with tenured positions, early in their professional career, and usually according to academic achievement tests" (Savelsberg 1994, 934-35). Most judges and prosecutors in the United States are either elected or nominated and confirmed through a political process that makes them more dependent on public approval and more vulnerable to political pressures (Savelsberg 1994). Another significant difference is that criminology is a core part of the law school curriculum in Germany. A large number of German law school students who are interested in criminal justice are familiar with the findings of empirical criminology. One leading German criminologist suggests that this might explain why German criminal judges "use the prison sentence in an essentially more reserved manner" than U.S. judges and overwhelmingly oppose the concept of deterrence via the death penalty (Pfeiffer 1996, 119). Criminal justice policy in Germany is also less vulnerable to political pres-

sures and radical shifts because academic experts are less dependant on policy-making institutions and political agencies for their funding (Savelsberg 1994).

The relative insulation and independence of the judiciary, criminal justice administrators, and academics are not the only institutional factors that explain why other Western countries are incarcerating people at low rates compared to the United States. Because of some important institutional changes recently, the U.S. criminal justice system has increased its capacity to absorb and process offenders and keep track of them on release. These changes have "enhanced the tendency for the system to drive its own growth" (Caplow and Simon 1999, 72). Ironically, the due process reforms of the 1960s and 1970s, which were intended to make the system fairer, have had some perverse effects, according to Caplow and Simon (1999). While these reforms have made the system more equitable in some important respects, they also have made it "more efficient with the result that it can be far more responsive to pressures for growth than it might have been in the past" (Caplow and Simon 1999, 98). For example, the state guarantee of the right to counsel for the poor may have improved the "overall capacity of the system to process cases efficiently" because defendants without legal representation often were "extremely difficult to manage" (Caplow and Simon 1999, 100). Numerous stories about the crushing caseloads of many public defenders today cast some doubt on their claim that the legal guarantee of the right to counsel has made it that much easier to process defendants through the system (see, e.g., Fritsch and Rhode 2001).

The due process revolution may have contributed in other ways to a tendency to incarcerate rather than dismiss charges or seek other, less severe sanctions. Before the 1970s, police and other correctional officers were not under any formal pressure to file charges quickly after rounding up a suspect. Thus, they were able to use "short-term jail time as a quasi-formal punishment." Now the authorities must decide early on whether to formally file charges. This "may in some cases result in a decision against arrest, but we suspect far more often it results in a decision to move forward" (Caplow and Simon 1999, 101). These are provocative suppositions about the due process revolution that Caplow and Simon (1999), in their broad-brush chapter, did not back up with hard data but that may merit further research.

Caplow and Simon (1999) did provide a detailed and convincing analysis of how changes in the institutions of parole and probation have enhanced the system's capacity to incarcerate. They and Joan Petersilia demonstrated how probation and parole, which once served as alternatives to imprisonment by providing supervision within the community, have become major sources of new prison admissions during the past two decades (Petersilia 1999, 479-529). Many offenders out on parole or probation are being sent back to prison for technical violations of the conditions of their release that are not actually crimes. Parole and probation officers routinely administer drug tests and are permitted to ignore the Fourth Amendment limitations on searches and seizures. Returns to prison are often accomplished using administrative procedures that do not include an automatic right to counsel and require a lower standard of proof than a court proceeding would. In 1991, 45 percent of prisoners had been on parole or probation before their current incarceration, compared to about 17 percent in 1974 (Caplow and Simon 1999, 102-103). Parole violators accounted for nearly two-thirds of all California prison admissions in 1997, and 41 percent of prison admissions were for violations of the technical conditions of parole rather than for convictions of new crimes (Austin and Lawson 1998, 483). Almost 700,000 parolees are now doing their time on U.S. streets. Most of them are supervised by parole systems that "provide few services and impose conditions that almost guarantee their failure," explained Petersilia (1999, 522-23). "Our monitoring systems are getting better, and public tolerance for failure on parole is decreasing. The result is that a rising tide of parolees is washing back into prison, putting pressures on states to build more prisons" (Petersilia 1999, 523).

Specific political context. It is important to understand how parole, probation, and the other institutional factors discussed above operate in a particular political context. The U.S. example is so striking not only because its overall incarceration rate is so much higher than other

Western countries' but also because of the enormous state-by-state variations in incarceration rates. One finds more diversity in the rates of imprisonment among the fifty states than when a comparison is drawn across the whole of Western Europe (Zimring and Hawkins 1991, chap. 6). While all states have seen an upward trend in their incarceration rates, there are still extreme variations between states. Texas and Louisiana, the most punitive states, incarcerate their citizens at about six times the rate of Minnesota and Maine, the least punitive.[18] California, which has the country's largest number of inmates (163,000) and operates the biggest penal system in the Western world, imprisons its population at the rate of 474 per 100,000, making it the twelfth most punitive state (Beck and Harrison 2001, Table 3:3).

Punishment and Democracy is a detailed study of how California's particular institutional and political context pushed the golden state's criminal justice policies in a sharply more punitive direction. California's version of three strikes is distinct because of "the extremity of its terms and the revolutionary nature of its ambitions" (Zimring, Hawkins, and Kamin 2001, ix). Penal populism as expressed through measures like three strikes is a national phenomenon, as is growing mistrust of the government. In a three-year period in the 1990s, twenty-six versions of three strikes legislation were enacted by states and the federal government. Nearly all of these measures were largely symbolic nods to penal populism and had only minimal impact on actual sentencing practices. Zimring and his coauthors attempted to explain why California's version of three strikes, which they described as the "largest penal experiment in American history," is far more severe and much larger in scope.[19]

Three strikes is really a misnomer for the California measure. Under the three strikes system there, defendants with only one residential burglary or violent conviction on their records who receive a second qualifying strike or conviction must be given prison terms double those mandated by the second offense. They also must serve a significantly larger fraction of their sentence prior to release. Together, these two provisions effectively triple the sentence for second-time offenders. Three strikes legislation in other jurisdictions requires two, not one, qualifying felonies before tougher sanctions are imposed. For defendants in California who have two prior qualifying offenses, a third felony conviction draws a mandatory twenty-five-years-to-life sentence. The federal government and many other states require that the third strike be for a serious felony conviction. But in California, the draconian third strike penalties are invoked even if the third felony conviction is something relatively mild like petty theft. California has generated more than 40,000 three strikes sentences. No other state has yet to generate 1,000, and the federal government has generated just 35 such sentences nationwide (Zimring, Hawkins, and Kamin 2001, 17-20).

Punishment and Democracy analyzes why three strikes measures elsewhere were designed to talk tough but have minimal impact, while the California version intentionally had the opposite effect. It identifies how institutional, historical, and political factors—and fate—intervened to buoy a measure that originated from marginal interest groups and initially did not have the backing of any powerful constituency in the legislature or executive branch. The October 1993 death of Polly Klaas, the twelve-year-old girl abducted from her home in a small town in Marin County and killed by a two-time violent offender, changed all that. Her death galvanized the movement to put a three strikes measure on California's November 1994 ballot. Up until then, the three strikes idea had been languishing in California and did not have any mainstream support. Facing reelection and saddled with an economic downturn, Republican Governor Pete Wilson seized on the law and order issue.

This helps explain why the legislature passed a three strikes bill in the spring of 1994 but not why it chose the most extreme of the five bills under consideration. First, California legislators had to contend with some powerful single-issue criminal justice lobbies, including the California Correctional Peace Officers Association (the prison guard union) and the National Rifle Association. As it became increasingly likely that voters would approve a three strikes measure on the November 1994 ballot, legislators sought to go on the offensive. Since Democrats did not want to hand Governor Wilson an issue for his reelection campaign,

they took an incredible gamble that backfired. Instead of choosing among the five alternatives, the legislative leadership backed itself into a corner by announcing in advance it would support whichever proposal Wilson chose. In but another example of how Democrats and liberal Republicans have been accomplices in the politics of penal populism, Willie Brown, the Democratic speaker of the California Assembly, "dared Governor Wilson, and the governor accepted that dare with a vengeance" (Zimring, Hawkins, and Kamin 2001, 12). In March 1994, Wilson announced his support for the harshest of the five alternatives and rejected a narrower bill submitted by the California District Attorneys Association. Legislators enacted the version Wilson selected without consulting with experts about either the drafting of the measure or its likely impact.

The immediate causes of California's "vulnerability to extreme versions of punitive law reform" (Zimring, Hawkins, and Kamin 2001, 170-71) were the Klaas tragedy, Wilson's electoral needs, and the Democrats' political gambit. A more fundamental institutional factor was the initiative process, which emboldens single-issue interest groups, encourages legislators to hastily preempt the normal legislative process, and discourages compromise (Zimring, Hawkins, and Kamin 2001). Another significant institutional factor was passage two decades earlier of the Determinate Sentencing Law. By stripping the parole boards of their authority, the 1976 law "removed a tradition of nonpolitical influence on time served" and created a precedent for politicizing the sentencing process (Zimring, Hawkins, and Kamin 2001, 172).

Zimring, Hawkins, and Kamin argued that the California outcome was highly contingent and unlikely to be replicated elsewhere. While other states are vulnerable to the sway of penal populism, California was particularly vulnerable because of the confluence of some exceptional factors, such as the initiative process and the commission of a particularly heinous crime just as the gubernatorial campaign was gearing up. "The breadth of the Three Strikes law [in California] was thus outside the range of legal changes that could ordinarily be expected to emerge from the political process," they concluded (Zimring, Hawkins, and Kamin 2001, 178).

Future trends. All of these works raise a related and more fundamental question about U.S. penal practices: is the race to incarcerate primarily a U.S. phenomenon or is it a harbinger of global trends? The fact that the incarceration rates of other countries continue to lag relatively far behind can reinforce the belief that the U.S. experience is distinct and likely to remain so. Yet a closer look at developments elsewhere casts some doubt on this. If Michael Tonry (cited in Frase 2001) is right that "America's today could be other countries' tomorrow," then it goes to say that "America's yesterday may be other countries' today," Frase suggested (p. 285).

Other Western countries are under increased pressure to take a more punitive stance because of several international developments, including growing fears about crossnational organized crime, drug trafficking, and illegal immigration, as well as changes at home (Morgan 2001, 384; Christie 1994; Mathiesen 1990, 1). The global war on terrorism in the aftermath of the 11 September attack on the World Trade Center has intensified the international pressure to move in a more punitive direction. While no country has made as fundamental a shift to a more repressive stance as the United States, some have taken steps in that direction. Even prior to 11 September, boot camps and zero tolerance were taking root in Australia, and the state of Victoria had responded to questionable opinion polls by implementing a wholesale increase in maximum penalties (Freiberg 2001, 53-54). The French Parliament recently enacted a new criminal code that provides for life imprisonment without parole. In England and Wales, life imprisonment has received new attention in the context of drug trafficking and violent and sexual offenses (Albrecht 2001, 303). With relatively little legislative encouragement, English courts have been steadily increasing their use of imprisonment. Between early 1993 and early 1997, England's prison population increased by 50 percent, a sudden, marked, and unprecedented expansion. According to the lord chief justice, the English judiciary was responding to what it perceived to be an increasingly punitive public mood (Ashworth 2001, 81-82).[20]

German criminal justice policy is no longer so insulated from public opinion and the electoral process. As a consequence, the "aspirations toward a more rational and humane sentencing policy and the rehabilitative optimism" that once characterized German sentencing policy may have run their course (Weigend 2001, 212). Crime statistics show that the level of serious crime in Germany has remained stable during the past decade despite the social upheavals brought about by reunification. Yet popular demands to toughen criminal sanctions are growing because of international crime, the pervasive belief in Germany that crime is on the rise, and the "lack of easily visible 'improvements' " in supposedly reformed offenders (Weigend 2001, 209). While Germany's sentencing practices remain moderate compared to other countries, German courts have demonstrated a new willingness to respond to the growing public fear of crime by imposing lengthy sentences. The German legislature also has passed some get-tough measures. Yet the new legislation has not sharply decreased judicial discretion, so sentencing courts retain the option of "adher[ing] to their own traditions oriented toward equitability and pragmatism" (Weigend 2001, 212).

The most dramatic change has been in the Netherlands, long recognized as one of the least punitive countries in the world. The incarceration rate there began rising steeply in the 1990s and is now 90 per 100,000, nearly five times what it was in the early 1970s.[21] The escalating crime rate, the increasing seriousness of criminal behavior, and broader changes in the political and academic culture help explain the

rise. Growing public concern that it was inhumane to have convicted offenders wait years before serving their sentences because of inadequate prison capacity also put pressure on the authorities to build more prisons.[22] Viewed as "the weak link in the mighty chain of international drugs [sic] control," the Netherlands also has faced intensified pressure from other countries to take a tough stance on drug-related crime (Downes 1988, 124-25). The 1988 United Nations Convention Against Drug Trafficking, the first major international agreement to standardize the approach to drugs, adopted a strongly punitive style modeled on the U.S. approach. It targets not just drug offenses but related problems, such as organized crime, corruption, and illegal profits, and it has propelled demands for wider powers for law enforcement in the Netherlands and other Western countries (Albrecht 2001, 300, 316-17; Frase 2001, 265).

Europe is not moving lockstep in a more punitive direction. There are some pulls the other way. The Dutch penal climate remains relatively mild. The Netherlands offers a range of alternatives to avoid imprisonment or shorten sentences, and Dutch prisons continue to be some of the most caring in the world. The Netherlands recently revised its prison policies to make its facilities more humane and to further limit the damaging effects of incarceration.[23] Norway and Portugal have abolished life imprisonment. The German constitutional court has ruled that life imprisonment must include the possibility of release (except for dangerous offenders), prompting the Parliament to amend the criminal code to allow parole in cases of life imprisonment after fifteen years for prisoners who do not present an ongoing threat to society (Albrecht 2001, 303). In several recent rulings, the European Court and Commission of Human Rights have taken some tentative steps toward establishing international standards for sentencing decisions that stress norms of proportionality (Kurki 2001, 331-78).

REVERSING THE BOOM IN THE UNITED STATES

With more than 2 million people sitting behind bars today and tens of millions more somehow enmeshed in the criminal justice system, the penal policies of the United States have a certain taken-for-granted quality. Just as it seemed unimaginable thirty years ago that the United States would be imprisoning its people at such unprecedented rates, today it seems almost unimaginable that the country will reverse course and begin to empty and board up its prisons. Yet, as Thomas Mathiesen (1990) reminded us, "Major repressive systems have succeeded in looking extremely stable almost until the day they have collapsed" (p. 167).

What is likely to reverse this trend? First, there is a need for more and better research. A number of the authors discussed here lamented the dearth of research in several areas related to criminal justice policy. Some went as far as to claim that politicians and government officials have intentionally locked the experts

out of the process to serve their own political needs.[24] These works are forays into several critical areas that remain largely unexplored, including comparative and historical scholarship on criminal justice, the implementation of specific penal policies, and the collateral consequences of incarceration.

Comparative and historical work. Policy makers, scholars, and activists need to pay more attention to documenting and explaining variations in sentencing and other penal practices across borders. To do so, they must begin by closing the comparative data gap. Cross-national statistics on crime rates, sentencing, and other aspects of criminal justice can be incomplete or misleading and thus vulnerable to charges of comparing apples with oranges. Frase (2001) contended that

until concrete, apples-with-apples data is available, skeptical U.S. citizens and their leaders will continue to ignore foreign comparisons, and observers both in and outside of the United States may misunderstand the true nature and extent of variations in sentencing between jurisdictions and over time within jurisdictions. (P. 284)

Policy makers, scholars, and activists also need to look more closely at the comparative history of various penal systems. Historical studies can serve several purposes. First, studying a system over time helps illuminate the relative significance or insignificance of political culture in explaining certain penal developments. Taking the long historical view also sensitizes us to the broad similarities in the evolution of penal systems. It reminds us that the policies of mass incarceration that the United States has pursued during the past three decades may be harbingers of penal developments elsewhere. Historical studies, like cross-national ones, can also be an important source of new ideas. Furthermore, they are a potent reminder that "old ideas" have "a way of coming back periodically, even when we do not recognize them as 'reruns'" (Frase 2001, 285).

Policy implementation. Another conspicuous research gap is the lack of detailed studies of how specific penal policies and programs are actually implemented. Ann Chih Lin's *Reform in the Making* and Zimring, Hawkins, and Kamin's *Punishment and Democracy* are important exceptions. *Reform in the Making*, which is based on hundreds of interviews with prison administrators, staff, and inmates and observation of classes, meetings, and other prison activities examines the fate of rehabilitative programs in five medium-security prisons in the United States. Lin argued that the rehabilitative ideal was discredited and discarded without ever really having been given a fair hearing. Lin showed how identical programs will have vastly different effects on the ground depending on how prisons vary in their institutional need for order and the institutional values that govern their different strategies for maintaining order. Lin faulted researchers and policy makers for their tendency to view programs in isolation, separate from the specific organizational environment of the correctional facilities charged with implementing them. "Every grand idea and good wish that policy-makers have lies in the hands of others," she explained (p. 14).

The largest multistate qualitative study of prisons in the United States, *Reform in the Making* masterfully uses survey, interview, and participant-observation techniques. In the appendixes, Lin elaborated on her methodology and discussed some of the key decisions she made along the way. She also discussed essential issues like establishing credibility and understanding bias. These appendixes should be required reading for any graduate student contemplating field research behind bars or in some equally foreign terrain.

Reform in the Making examines the complex and subtle ways that rehabilitative programs not only receive different levels of support in various prisons but also are understood differently in different prisons. Prisons that have successfully implemented literacy and other educational programs have staff members and inmates who believe that the programs serve their institutional needs and view the programs' rehabilitative goals and the prison's overall goals as complementary. While Lin did a good job at showing how institutional attitudes and values vary from prison to prison, it is less clear why they vary. She indicated that differences in the attitudes of the upper-level administrators and in the institutional history of the facilities help explain why the values and attitudes of prison staffs vary so decisively between prisons. One wonders whether differences in local and state-level politics are also important factors. It is difficult to gauge this from Lin's account. Like many researchers who have been granted wide access to prisons, Lin was forced to conceal the actual names and locales of the five facilities she studied. This prevented her from considering what effect the specific political environment had on each of the prisons she visited.

Lin discovered some success stories where they were least expected. "Beaverton," the prison in her sample with the highest percentage of inmates with violent histories, was relatively effective at implementation compared to some other prisons with less violent populations. At that federal institution, a high percentage of the prisoners signed up for the educational programs. During her visits to Beaverton's classrooms, Lin saw inmates "out of their seats, clustered in groups of four around tables with sheets of scrap paper, animatedly arguing about math formulas" (pp. 15-16). At a relatively unsuccessful prison, numerous educational and training programs existed on paper, but the teaching staff was embittered and isolated. Prisoners were reluctant to sign up for programs or were unaware of their existence. Sleeping or staring blankly ahead were common classroom activities. Implementation of the programs was essentially abandoned.

Unfortunately, the programs mandated at most prisons are carried out in ways that defeat their purposes. "The result is cynicism, not only about prisoners and their chances for reform, but about our capacity as a society to do more than put prisoners away and hope they stay gone," Lin argued (p. 17). She made a persuasive case that the rehabilitative ideal was buried without ever having been given a real chance.

Whether specific policies are effective at reintegrating prisoners into society is an important question. But no answer to it can be found if the policies in question are never implemented, do not function as designed, or are changed beyond recognition. (Lin 2000, 10-11)

"Before it is possible to test 'what works?' one must ensure that the conditions for a fair test exist" (Lin 2000, 10-11).

Zimring, Hawkins, and Kamin reached some equally surprising conclusions about the implementation of three strikes across California. By restricting judicial discretion, the measure ended up enhancing the discretion of prosecutors, relatively speaking. Prosecutors were much more likely to pursue second strike penalties, which were less dramatic departures from prior practice, than to invoke the draconian penalties for third strike offenders (p. 145). There were also wide geographical variations in implementation. San Francisco prosecutors were much less likely to invoke the penalties outlined in three strikes than were prosecuting attorneys in San Diego (pp. 218-19). While the three strikes measure put substantial additional pressure on courts to process cases, "the trial crunch fell far short of the system-paralyzing seriousness that some had projected" because of an increase in prosecutorial plea-bargaining concessions in two strike cases and highly selective enforcement in eligible three strike cases (pp. 125-26). For these reasons, early predictions that the state's prison population would double within five years after passage of three strikes turned out to be widely off the mark. Zimring, Hawkins, and Kamin calculated that during the short term, the law has been responsible for less than a 10 percent net increase in California's prison population (pp. 134, 220). However, they did warn that if current prosecutorial trends continue, the law will result in a "steady stream of very long prison sentences" that "will be leaving a residue of additional prisoners behind bars for much longer terms, and this process will reach its maximum impact 15 and 20 years after 1994" (p. 146). That forecast looks more uncertain in the aftermath of a federal appeals court decision in November 2001 that threw out a shoplifter's fifty-year sentence under California's three strikes statute. The court ruled that the sentence violated the Constitution's ban on cruel and unusual punishment. This decision could result in hundreds of new appeals from defendants sentenced to long prison terms for petty crimes (Associated Press 2001, A-8).

Collateral consequences of prison. If the terms of the debate about prisons and crime are to change in the United States, there has to be a better understanding not only of implementation but also of the broader consequences of incarceration. Prisons mark not just the person who serves time but his or her family, his or her community, and the wider soci-

ety. For all the billions spent on prisons, so far there has been relatively little systematic attention to what John Hagan and Ronit Dinovitzer (1999) called the "collateral consequences" of prisons (pp. 121-162). Alison Liebling (1999), an expert on prison suicide, suggested that the "pains of imprisonment are basically underestimated," perhaps because they are awkward challenges to the belief that "prison works" (pp. 341-42). Many significant questions go largely unaddressed. Why do former prisoners have such reduced incomes and employment rates?[25] How does having a mother or father in prison affect the estimated 1.5 million children with an incarcerated parent? Susan Phillips and Barbara Bloom (cited in Hagan and Dinovitzer 1999, 138) suggested that by getting tough on crime, the United States has also gotten tough on the millions of children who will have a parent in prison at some point during their lifetimes. Another understudied question is, Why are the homicide and suicide rates in U.S. correctional facilities so high (Bottoms 1999, 205-81; Liebling 1999, 283-359)? And finally, what will happen to the distribution of health care resources in prisons and the wider society as prisons increasingly house a disproportionate number of people with substance abuse, mental illnesses, and infectious diseases such as HIV, tuberculosis, and hepatitis C and as more inmates grow old behind bars (McDonald 1999, 427-78)?

Experts and activists need to figure out how to make prisons and the lives they mark more visible to the wider society. In the nineteenth century, prisons opened their doors to the public and were a popular destination for gawking domestic and foreign tourists. In the 1960s and early 1970s, prison memoirs and accounts of life behind bars turned up occasionally on best-seller lists. Today, prisons are a mystery. "Prisons are all around us but we choose not to notice, and more than we admit, perhaps more than we realize, so-called corrections is a central feature of American society," explained one historian of incarceration (Christianson 1998, ix). *Going up the River* and *Reform in the Making* do a particularly good job of making life in prison real and visible. They complement each other, for Hallinan focused on some of the most brutal practices at maximum-security institutions and Lin examined medium-security facilities.

Hallinan's book is short on analysis. What analysis there is tends to be superficial. In several places, Hallinan made claims that are either unsubstantiated or at odds with generally accepted research. That said, the book is valuable because it contains rich, vivid, and disturbing vignettes of life in prison and in the incarceral communities that have grown up around correctional facilities. Hallinan described a visit to a penal farm in Beeville, Texas, where convicts, many of them African American, do backbreaking work as field hands. As they pound the earth in the blazing sun, the inmates sing songs handed down by convicts from generation to generation. Some of the songs date back to the antebellum era. Trailed by packs of hounds, armed guards on horseback watch over the inmates, who address the guards as "Boss," as in "Boss Jones," in another convention dating from the plantation era (pp. 4, 13). The bosses carry .357 Magnums and are authorized to shoot to kill. Hallinan described other antiquated practices. In Alabama, the state continued to chain misbehaving inmates to hitching posts until 1998, something no state had done for a quarter of a century. The practice stopped only after a federal judge ruled it unconstitutional. Alabama still continues the practice of forcing inmates caught masturbating to wear special flamingo pink uniforms (p. 102). Oklahoma and Louisiana still host prison rodeos. The main event at the annual McAlester, Oklahoma, rodeo is Money the Hard Way. A tobacco sack is tied between the horns of a bull, and the bull is then released into an arena with several dozen inmates. The first inmate bold enough to grab the sack wins at least $100, which equals about five months of prison pay. On a Saturday night, the rodeo can attract upwards of ten thousand people. The rodeo earns tens of thousands of dollars for the prison and the local chamber of commerce, which helps run it (pp. 187, 197). *Going up the River* also includes gripping and chilling descriptions of death row, administrative segregation, and the new supermax facilities, where offenders are kept nearly around the clock in windowless, spartan cells designed to eliminate virtually all human contact and interaction.[26]

Reform in the Making avoids some of the pitfalls of both scholarly and popular works on incarceration.

Hallinan's portrait of prison is skewed to the extremes—penal farms in Texas; death row in McAlester, Oklahoma; the Security Housing Unit in Pelican Bay, California—and confirms the view of prison as a Hobbesian world. By contrast, Lin challenged the popular view of prisons as primarily "combat zones" where sadistic staff beat up "on vicious criminals, guns at the ready to face homemade but deadly knives and clubs" (p. 143). While danger is always present in the five medium-security facilities she studied, it is mostly "a backdrop for the mundane daily tasks of checking passes, getting the food served, and making sure that prisoners are where they are supposed to be," according to Lin (p. 34). Unlike many scholarly works that focus on prison management or the broader issue of public administration, Lin's does not treat the inmates as just one more task, input, or product to be managed. She included extensive direct quotations from inmates that poignantly capture the "seesaw between determination and disappointment" that rules their lives, especially as they contemplate life on the outside. Lin showed how the can-do spirit and force of will that many rehabilitative programs try to inculcate in prisoners can evaporate in the face of barriers over which inmates have little control. One inmate's description of his despair and anger after being turned down for a supermarket job in a predominantly white town once the manager discovered he was black is heartbreaking (p. 143). Lin chided many rehabilitative programs for stressing to inmates how, on release,

if they have the will and skill, they will reach their goals, however lofty or mundane. She argued that prison programs need to give inmates room to lower their expectations and construct goals that will not leave them disappointed. Rehabilitative programs also need to more directly acknowledge to inmates the barriers they face that are not of their own making, such as racial prejudice and the widespread reluctance to hire ex-offenders (p. 144).

Role of the experts. More and better research on prisons and making prisons visible again to the wider society are important first steps toward reversing the race to incarcerate. Zimring, Hawkins, and Kamin went a step further and argued that the experts may hold the key to changing the politics of crime and punishment in the United States. They contended that the country needs to figure out how to return criminal policy once again to the experts by creating institutions that are insulated from the politicians and the public. Their model is the U.S. Federal Reserve. "The lesson here for criminal justice reform is the importance of a commitment and respect for expertise, which is itself a justifying ideology for the insulated delegation of punishment power" (p. 209). They suggested that sentencing commissions, if properly constructed, might serve as a model of insulated delegation for criminal justice policy analogous to what the Federal Reserve does for monetary policy (pp. 212-14).

Zimring, Hawkins, and Kamin did not specify the political preconditions that would be necessary to create such insulated institutions. They did concede that the conditions necessary to create institutions insulated from democratic review, and those necessary to maintain those institutions once they are up and running, are not the same. One can infer from their analysis that they do not expect the public, with its anti-offender sentiments, to play a constructive role here. Yet *Punishment and Democracy* may be guilty of expecting too much from the experts and too little from the public. In stressing the potentially constructive role that experts can play in penal policy, one has to keep in mind that the so-called experts have been responsible for some diabolical penal practices in the past. In his brief chapter on how the scientific experts replaced the moralists as the guiding force in prison reform more than a century ago, Hallinan briefly surveyed the checkered history of the experts in penal reform. Over the years, the experts have subjected inmates to therapies ranging from the relatively harmless, like bibliotherapy, to the bizarre and dangerous, like testicular implantation.[27]

Zimring, Hawkins, and Kamin may have taken too harsh and skeptical a view of the public. As mentioned earlier, polls consistently indicate that U.S. public opinion on criminal justice is fickle and highly malleable in the face of specific events and political manipulation. Moreover, there is some evidence that penal populism may be peaking. In the 2000 elections, measures to soften drug laws were on the ballots of seven states, and voters approved

five of them. The best known of these initiatives was Proposition 36 in California. Passed by an overwhelming majority, it requires treatment instead of jail for drug offenders and calls for providing treatment rather than a return to prison for parolees who test positive for drugs (Muwakkil 2000, 25-26). A record number of measures to soften drug laws are pending or have been passed by state legislatures during the past year (Turner 2001). Recent national debates over high-profile death penalty cases (most notably the execution of Timothy McVeigh for the Oklahoma City bombing) and over the execution of juveniles and the mentally retarded indicate some softening of public sentiment on capital punishment.

Political leadership. If the comparative history of incarceration teaches us anything, it is that political leadership, not expertise alone, has been responsible for major decarcerations elsewhere. But politicians have to be pushed, sometimes by the public, sometimes by the experts. In Finland, the small group of experts involved in criminal justice in the 1960s and 1970s became convinced that Finland's high incarceration rate was a disgrace. They provided the data to demonstrate that Finland's imprisonment rate was way out of line with other European countries and unrelated to the level of crime. They reached out to the politicians, civil servants, and public by arguing that criminal justice policy had to be seen in a wider societal context that stressed not only the costs of criminality but also the costs in monetary and human terms of controlling crime. That view was captured by their slogan, "Criminal policy is an inseparable part of social development policy" (Lappi-Seppälä 2001, 108; Törnudd 1997). In rare instances, politicians are moved to act by strong personal beliefs about right and wrong. Early in the twentieth century, England underwent a major decarceration, prompted in large part by Winston Churchill. During his brief tenure as home secretary, Churchill expressed deep skepticism about what could be achieved through incarceration and quickly came to believe the prison system was overused (Rutherford 1986, 124). Churchill once said, "The mood and temper of the public in regard to the treatment of crime and criminals is one of the most unfailing tests of the civilization of any country" (Garland 1990, 215). The really interesting and pressing question is not whether the experts, the politicians, or the public is going to lead the United States out of its incarceration mess but rather how you fashion an effective coalition from members of all three groups to begin emptying the country's prisons.

MARIE GOTTSCHALK

Notes

1. There were some significant fluctuations during this period, notably during the Depression. See Cahalan (1979).

2. Prisons usually are state facilities that confine long-term offenders convicted of felonies. Jails generally are county and city facilities that house people awaiting trial, offenders convicted of misdemeanors, and short-term felony offenders.

3. For a good discussion of how studies of comparative prison use are fraught with possibilities for misinterpretation, see Pease (1994) and Young and Brown (1993).

4. The 11 September attack on the World Trade Center resulted in an upsurge in public confidence in the government that defied historic trends (see Stille 2001, A-13).

5. For example, the proportion of Gallup-poll respondents who agreed that crime or violence "is the most important problem facing this country today" varied from 1 to 6 percent between 1982 and 1992, was 9 percent in January 1993, and then jumped to 37 percent and 52 percent, respectively, in January and August 1994 in the months leading up to enactment of a massive crime bill supported by President Bill Clinton (Bureau of Justice Statistics, cited in Frase 2001, 268).

6. For a subtle analysis of the growing gap between elite and mass public opinion and the increased willingness of politicians to use "crafted talk" to manipulate mass public opinion to their advantage, see Jacobs and Shapiro (2000).

7. For an excellent discussion of how identity politics as expressed through hate crimes legislation has distorted the discourse about crime in the United States, see Jacobs and Potter (1998).

8. Erikson (1966) did not characterize the Quaker persecutions and Salem witch trials he analyzed as "moral panics." The term was not in use yet. Building on Durkheim's work, he viewed these events as "crime waves" that were useful for identifying and demarcating acceptable and unacceptable behavior and thus knitting the community more tightly together.

9. For more on the U.S. Congress and drug policy in the early years of the Nixon administration, see Peterson (1985).

10. On Rockefeller, Nixon, and the war on drugs, see Massing (1998, 126-29) and Epstein (1977, chap. 2).

11. The results of the University of Michigan annual survey of high school drug use released in January 1994 showed the first increase in marijuana use in fourteen years. This rise prompted the Clinton administration to stake out a more hard-line position on

drugs, even though marijuana use was still less than half what it had been in the late 1970s and consumption of hard drugs remained negligible (Massing 1998, 213-19).

12. The Corrections Corporation of America's stock subsequently plummeted (see Hallinan 2001, 184).

13. Grace Defina of the Concerned Citizens of Wayne County, Pennsylvania, which is battling the construction of a prison in her community, made similar points at the workshop.

14. An example is the conference Critical Resistance East: Beyond the Prison Industrial Complex, at Columbia University Law School, 9-11 March 2001, organized by the Critical Northeast Regional Organizing Committee.

15. For an excellent discussion of how this works in practice, see Doob (1995).

16. Wilson (cited in Reitz 2001), once a fierce proponent of the incapacitative effects of prison, subsequently conceded that "very large increases in the prison population can produce only modest reductions in crime rates" (p. 236).

17. The rehabilitative ideal is the belief that prisons could serve to rehabilitate offenders (see Allen 1981).

18. The rate for Louisiana is 801 per 100,000. Texas is 730 per 100,000. Minnesota and Maine are, respectively, 129 and 128 per 100,000. The highest rate in the nation is technically the District of Columbia, with 971 per 100,000 (Beck and Harrison 2001, Table 3.3).

19. This is the title they give to chapter 2.

20. For more on England's turn toward harsher sanctions, see Rutherford (1986, 172) and Lewis (1997, 229).

21. The low numbers for the 1970s may have been misleading because they did not include all the people on the waiting list to be incarcerated (Tak 2001, 151).

22. Prison capacity there has quadrupled in the past two decades (Tak 2001, 179; see also Christie 1994).

23. Prisoners are no longer denied the right to vote, and each prisoner has some statutorily guaranteed activities, including open-air visits, visits by family and friends, recreation, and sports. Productive labor for twenty-six hours per week is also a central part of the new policy (Tak 2001, 184-85).

24. In 1999, for example, there was an intense legislative struggle in California over a proposal for a publicly funded study of three strikes. The chief sponsors of the measure were liberal Democratic legislators who were opposed to three strikes and wanted to build a case for weakening it. They eventually prevailed over supporters of three strikes, who did not want the presumed effectiveness of the legislation open to scrutiny (Zimring, Hawkins, and Kamin 2001, 220-21).

25. Some promising new work in this area includes Western and McLanahan (2000) and Western and Pettit (2000).

26. Supermax inmates lucky enough to receive counseling must speak to their therapists through a slit less than an inch wide that runs the length of each cell door. In this cell-front counseling, what the inmate says to the counselor is open to anyone within earshot, including guards and other inmates (Hallinan 2001, 208).

27. In this procedure, physicians removed the testicles from men who had just been executed, ground them into a substance the consistency of toothpaste, and injected them with a syringe into the abdomens of other inmates (Hallinan, 2001, 77).

References

Albrecht, Hans-Jörg. 2001. Post-adjudication dispositions in comparative perspective. In *Sentencing and sanctions in Western countries*, edited by Michael Tonry and Richard S. Frase. Oxford, UK: Oxford University Press.

Allen, Francis. 1981. *The decline of the rehabilitative ideal*. New Haven, CT: Yale University Press.

Ashworth, Andrew. 2001. The decline of English sentencing and other stories. In *Sentencing and sanctions in Western countries*, edited by Michael Tonry and Richard S. Frase. Oxford, UK: Oxford University Press.

Associated Press. 2001. Court rejects 3-strikes term for shoplifter. *New York Times*, 3 November, A-8.

Austin, James, and Robert Lawson. 1998. Assessment of California parole violations and recommended intermediate programs and policies. In *Parole and prisoner reentry in the United States*, edited by Joan Petersilia. San Francisco: National Council on Crime and Delinquency.

Beck, Allen J., and Paige M. Harrison. 2001. Prisoners in 2000. *Bureau of Justice Statistics Bulletin*, no. NCJ 188207 (August): 1-15.

Berke, Richard L., and Janet Elder. 2001. Bush loses favor despite tax cut and overseas trip. *New York Times*, 21 June, A-1.

Blumstein, Alfred, and Allen J. Beck. 1999. Population growth in U.S. prisons, 1980-1996. In *Prisons: Crime and justice—A review of research*, vol. 26, edited by Michael Tonry and Joan Petersilia. Chicago: University of Chicago Press.

Bottoms, Anthony E. 1999. Interpersonal violence and social order in prisons. In *Prisons: Crime and justice—A review of research*, vol. 26, edited by Michael Tonry and Joan Petersilia. Chicago: University of Chicago Press.

Cahalan, Margaret. 1979. Trends in incarceration in the United States since 1980: A summary of reported rates and the distribution of officers. *Crime & Delinquency* 25(1):9-41.

Caplow, Theodore, and Jonathan Simon. 1999. Understanding prison policy and population trends. In *Prisons: Crime and justice—A review of research*, vol. 26, edited by Michael Tonry and Joan Petersilia. Chicago: University of Chicago Press.

Chesney-Lind, Meda. 1988. Women in prison: From partial justice to vengeful equity. *Corrections Today* 60 (7): 66-73.

Christianson, Scott. 1998. *With liberty for some: 500 years of imprisonment in America*. Boston: Northeastern University Press.

Christie, Nils. 1994. *Crime control as industry: Toward GULAGS, Western style*. 2d ed. London: Routledge.

Currie, Elliott. 1985. *Confronting crime: An American challenge*. New York: Pantheon.

———. 1998. *Crime and punishment in America*. New York: Metropolitan Books.

Doob, Anthony. 1995. The United States sentencing commission guidelines: If you don't know where you are going, you might not get there. In *The politics of sentencing reform*, edited by Chris Clarkson and Rod Morgan. Oxford, UK: Clarendon-Oxford University Press.

Downes, David. 1988. *Contrasts in tolerance: Post-war penal policy in the Netherlands and England and Wales*. Oxford, UK: Clarendon.

Epstein, Edward Jay. 1977. *Agency of fear: Opiates and political power in America*. New York: G. P. Putnam.

Erikson, Kai T. 1966. *Wayward Puritans: A study in the sociology of deviance*. New York: John Wiley.

Feeley, Malcolm M., and Jonathan Simon. 1992. The new penology: Notes on the emerging strategy of corrections and its implications. *Criminology* 30 (4): 449-74.

Frase, Richard S. 2001. Comparative perspectives in sentencing policy and research. In *Sentencing and sanctions in Western countries*, edited by Michael Tonry and Richard S. Frase. Oxford, UK: Oxford University Press.

Freiberg, Arie. 2001. Three strikes and you're out—It's not cricket: Colonization and resistance in Australian sentencing. In *Sentencing and sanctions in Western countries*, edited by Michael Tonry and Richard S. Frase. Oxford, UK: Oxford University Press.

Friedman, Lawrence M. 1993. *Crime and punishment in American history*. New York: Basic Books.

Fritsch, Jane, and David Rhode. 2001. Two-tier justice. *New York Times*, 8-10 April.

Garland, David. 1990. *Punishment and modern society: A study in social theory*. Chicago: Chicago University Press.

————. 2001. *The culture of control: Social order in contemporary society.* Chicago: University of Chicago Press.

Gilmore, Craig. 2001. Remarks presented at Prisons in Rural America: Overview for Social Change Activists, at Critical Resistance East: Beyond the Prison Industrial Complex, Critical Northeast Regional Organizing Committee, Columbia University Law School, New York, 10 March.

Gilmore, Ruth Wilson. 2001. Remarks presented at Prisons in Rural America: Overview for Social Change Activists, at Critical Resistance East: Beyond the Prison Industrial Complex, Critical Northeast Regional Organizing Committee, Columbia University Law School, New York, 10 March.

Gonnerman, Jennifer. 2000. Two million and counting. *Village Voice*, 22 February, 56.

Hagan, John, and Ronit Dinovitzer. 1999. Collateral consequences of imprisonment for children, communities, and prisoners. In *Prisons: Crime and justice—A review of research*, vol. 26, edited by Michael Tonry and Joan Petersilia. Chicago: University of Chicago Press.

Harwood, John, and Jeanne Cummings. 2001. Bush's approval rating slips to 50%, a 5-year presidential low. *Wall Street Journal*, 28 June, A-18.

Jacobs, James B., and Kimberly Potter. 1998. *Hate crimes: Criminal law and identity politics.* New York: Oxford University Press.

Jacobs, Lawrence R., and Robert Y. Shapiro. 2000. *Politicians don't pander: Political manipulation and the loss of democratic responsiveness.* Chicago: University of Chicago Press.

Kurki, Leena. 2001. International standards for sentencing and punishment. In *Sentencing and sanctions in Western countries*, edited by Michael Tonry and Richard S. Frase. Oxford, UK: Oxford University Press.

Lappi-Seppälä, Tapio. 2001. Sentencing and punishment in Finland: The decline of the repressive ideal. In *Sentencing and sanctions in Western countries*, edited by Michael Tonry and Richard S. Frase. Oxford, UK: Oxford University Press.

Lewis, Derek. 1997. *Hidden agendas: Politics, law and disorder.* London: Hamish Hamilton.

Liebling, Alison. 1999. Prison suicide and prisoner coping. In *Prisons: Crime and justice—A review of research*, vol. 26, edited by Michael Tonry and Joan Petersilia. Chicago: University of Chicago Press.

Massing, Michael. 1998. *The fix.* New York: Simon & Schuster.

Mathiesen, Thomas. 1990. *Prison on trial: A critical assessment.* London: Sage.

McDonald, Douglas C. 1999. Medical care in prisons. In *Prisons: Crime and justice—A review of research*, vol. 26, edited by Michael Tonry and Joan Petersilia. Chicago: University of Chicago Press.

Morgan, Rod. 2001. International controls in sentencing and sanctions. In *Sentencing and sanctions in Western countries*, edited by Michael Tonry and Richard S. Frase. Oxford, UK: Oxford University Press.

Muwakkil, Salim. 2000. Just vote no: The war on drugs loses at the polls. *In These Times*, 25 December, 25-26.

Pease, Ken. 1994. Cross-national imprisonment rates. *British Journal of Criminology* 34: 116-30.

Petersilia, Joan. 1999. Parole and prisoner reentry in the United States. In *Prisons: Crime and justice—A review of research*, vol. 26, edited by Michael Tonry and Joan Petersilia. Chicago: University of Chicago Press.

Peterson, Ruth D. 1985. Discriminatory decision making at the legislative level: An analysis of the Comprehensive Drug Abuse Prevention and Control Act of 1970. *Law and Human Behavior* 9 (3): 243-69.

Pfeiffer, Christian. 1996. Crisis in American criminal policy? A letter to Mrs. J. Reno, attorney general of the United States of America. *European Journal on Criminal Policy and Research* 4 (2): 118-27.

Pollock-Byrne, M. 1990. *Women, prison, crime*. Pacific Grove, CA: Brooks/Cole.

Reitz, Kevin R. 2001. The disassembly and reassembly of U.S. sentencing practices. In *Sentencing and sanctions in Western countries*, edited by Michael Tonry and Richard S. Frase. Oxford, UK: Oxford University Press.

Rutherford, Andrew. 1986. *Prisons and the process of justice: The reductionist challenge*. London: Heinemann.

Savelsberg, Joachim J. 1994. Knowledge, domination, and criminal punishment. *American Journal of Sociology* 99 (4): 911-43.

Stille, Alexander. 2001. Suddenly, Americans trust Uncle Sam. *New York Times*, 3 November, A-13.

Stith, Kate, and Steve Y. Koh. 1993. The politics of sentencing reform: The legislative history of the federal sentencing guidelines. *Wake Forest Law Review* 28 (2): 223-90.

Tak, Peter J. 2001. Sentencing and punishment in the Netherlands. In *Sentencing and sanctions in Western countries*, edited by Michael Tonry and Richard S. Frase. Oxford, UK: Oxford University Press.

Talvi, Silja J. A. 2001. Women behind bars. *Prison Legal News* 12 (6): 1-4.

Tonry, Michael. 1995. *Malign neglect: Race, crime and punishment in America*. New York: Oxford University Press.

———. 2001. Punishment policies and patterns in Western countries. In *Sentencing and sanctions in Western countries*, edited by Michael Tonry and Richard S. Frase. Oxford, UK: Oxford University Press.

Tonry, Michael, and Joan Petersilia. 1999. American prisons at the beginning of the twenty-first century. In *Prisons: Crime and justice—A review of research*, vol. 26, edited by Michael Tonry and Joan Petersilia. Chicago: University of Chicago Press.

Törnudd, Patrik. 1997. Sentencing and punishment in Finland. In *Sentencing reform in overcrowded times: A comparative perspective*, edited by Michael Tonry and Kathleen Hatlestad. New York: Oxford University Press.

Turner, Nicholas R. 2001. Paper presented at the annual meeting of the American Correctional Association. Sensible sentencing: Structured sentencing and sentencing reform, Philadelphia, 15 August.

von Hirsch, Andrew. 2001. The project of sentencing reform. In *Sentencing and sanctions in Western countries*, edited by Michael Tonry and Richard S. Frase. Oxford, UK: Oxford University Press.

Weigend, Thomas. 2001. Sentencing and punishment in Germany. In *Sentencing and sanctions in Western countries*, edited by Michael Tonry and Richard S. Frase. Oxford, UK: Oxford University Press.

Western, Bruce, and Sara McLanahan. 2000. Fathers behind bars: The impact of incarceration on family formation. In *Families, crime and criminal justice: Charting the linkages*. Greenwich, CT: JAI/Elsevier.

Western, Bruce, and Becky Pettit. 2000. Incarceration and racial inequality in men's employment. *Industrial and Labor Relations Review* 54 (1): 3-16.

Wilson, James Q. 1975. *Thinking about crime*. New York: Basic Books.

Young, Warren, and Mark Brown. 1993. Cross-national comparisons of imprisonment. In *Crime and justice: A review of research*, vol. 17, edited by Michael Tonry. Chicago: University of Chicago Press, 1-49.

Zimring, Franklin E. 2000. Imprisonment rates and the new politics of criminal punishment. Paper presented at The causes and consequences of mass imprisonment in the USA conference, New York University School of Law, 26 February.

———. 2001. Imprisonment rates and the new politics of criminal punishment. *Punishment and Society* 3 (1): 161-66.

Zimring, Franklin E., and Gordon Hawkins. 1991. *The scale of imprisonment.* Chicago: University of Chicago Press.

———. 1995. *Incapacitation.* New York: Oxford University Press.

Erratum

In the March 2002 issue of *The Annals*, Figure 1 was printed incorrectly in the article "The Transition to Adulthood: A Time Use Perspective," authored by Anne H. Gauthier and Frank F. Furstenberg Jr. The correct figure appears here.

FIGURE 1
TIME SPENT ON VARIOUS ACTIVITIES BY YOUNG ADULTS AGES 18 TO 34, BY GENDER, TRANSITION STATUS, AND COUNTRY

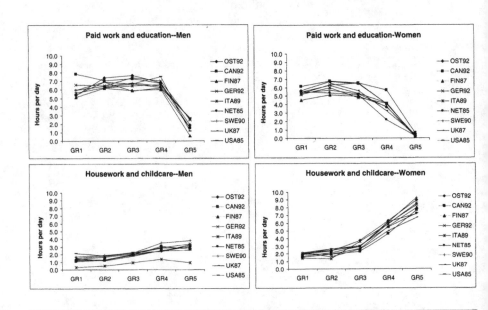

FIGURE 1 Continued

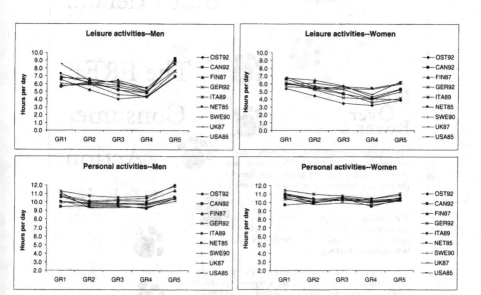

NOTES: OST92 = Austria (1992); CAN92 = Canada (1992); FIN87 = Finland (1987); GER92 = Germany (1992); ITA89 = Italy (1989); NET85 = Netherlands (1985); SWE90 = Sweden (1990); UK87 = United Kingdom (1987); USA85 = United States (1985); GR1 = nonpartnered students without children; GR2 = nonpartnered employed people without children; GR3 = partnered employed people without children; GR4 = partnered employed people with children under age fifteen; GR5 = nonemployed people (and not students) with and without children (for men) and with children (for women). All results based on weighted data.

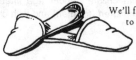

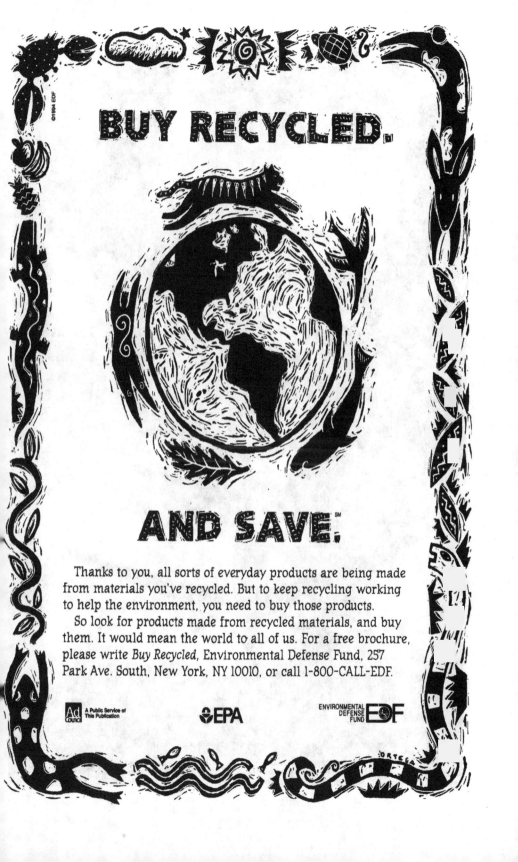

You aren't looking at
a future pilot.

You're looking at YOUR
future pilot.

Higher academic standards are good for everyone.
What a child learns today could have a major effect tomorrow. Not just on him or her, but on the rest of
the world. Your world. Since 1992, we've worked to raise academic standards. Because quite simply,
smarter kids make smarter adults. For more information, call 1-800-38-BE-SMART or visit www.edex.org.

The Business Roundtable • U.S. Department of Education • Achieve
American Federation of Teachers • National Alliance of Business
National Education Association • National Governors' Association

Education Excellence Partnership

Printed in the United States
By Bookmasters

Printed in the United States
By Bookmasters